American Cancer Society's

Guide to

Pain
Control

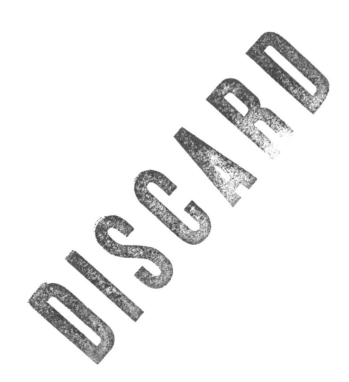

BOOKS PUBLISHED BY THE AMERICAN CANCER SOCIETY

A Breast Cancer Journey: Your Personal Guidebook

American Cancer Society's Guide to Complementary and Alternative Cancer Methods

Cancer in the Family: Helping Children Cope with a Parent's Illness, Heiney et al.

Caregiving: A Step-By-Step Resource for Caring for the Person with Cancer at Home, Houts and Bucher

Colorectal Cancer: A Thorough and Compassionate Resource for Patients and Their Families, Levin

Consumers Guide to Cancer Drugs, Wilkes et al.

Informed Decisions: The Complete Book of Cancer Diagnosis, Treatment, and Recovery, Second Edition, Eyre et al.

Our Mom Has Cancer, Ackermann and Ackermann

Prostate Cancer: What Every Man—and His Family—Needs to Know, Revised Edition, Bostwick et al.

Women and Cancer: A Thorough and Compassionate Resource for Patients and Their Families, Runowicz et al.

ALSO BY THE AMERICAN CANCER SOCIETY

American Cancer Society's Healthy Eating Cookbook: A Celebration of Food, Friends, and Healthy Living, Second Edition

Celebrate! Healthy Entertaining for Any Occasion

Kids' First Cookbook: Delicious-Nutritious Treats to Make Yourself!

American Cancer Society's

Guide to

Pain Control

Powerful Methods to Overcome Cancer Pain

Published by
American Cancer Society
Health Content Products
1599 Clifton Road NE
Atlanta, Georgia 30329, USA

Printed in the United States of America
Designed by Jill Dible
Cover designed by Barbara Werden

5 4 3 2 1   01 02 03 04 05

Library of Congress Cataloging-in-Publication Data

Guide to pain control
    American Cancer Society's guide to pain control
        p. cm.
    Includes index.
    ISBN 0-944235-33-6
      1.   Cancer pain. I. American Cancer Society.

  RC262.G788 2001
  616'.0472—dc21

                                                                        2001022496

A Note to the Reader
The information contained in this book is not intended as medical advice and should not be relied upon as a substitute for consulting with your physician. This information may not address all possible actions, precautions, side effects, or interactions. All matters regarding your health require the supervision of a physician who is familiar with your medical needs. For more information, contact your American Cancer Society at 1-800-ACS-2345 (www.cancer.org).

American Cancer Society's

Guide to

Pain Control

Managing Editor
Katherine V. Bruss, Psy.D.

Contributors
Steve Frandzel
Esmeralda Galán
Amy Sproull
Leah Tuzzio

Editorial Review
Betty R. Ferrell, Ph.D., F.A.A.N.
Research Scientist
City of Hope National Medical Center
Duarte, California

Terri B. Ades, R.N., M.S., A.O.C.N.
Rick Alteri, M.D.
Joy L. Fincannon, R.N., M.S.
Karen Russell, R.N., M.S.N., O.C.N.

Publishing Director
Emily Pualwan

Production Manager
Candace Magee

Contents

Foreword

by Betty R. Ferrell, Ph.D., F.A.A.N.
Research Scientist, City of Hope National Medical Center

The American Cancer Society is dedicated to enhancing the quality of life for individuals facing cancer across the cancer journey including attention before diagnosis, initial treatment, survivorship, recurrence, and care at the end-of-life. There is no aspect of cancer that is so overwhelming for both patients and families and has the ability to diminish quality of life than the problem of pain. Pain consumes the patient experiencing it and is perhaps even worse for family members who must observe pain in someone they love. Pain is an all-consuming experience including dimensions of physical, psychological, social, and spiritual well being.

In the 1990s, there was increased attention focused on the problem of pain by health care professionals. Numerous organizations, including the American Cancer Society, the World Health Organization, federal agencies, and other national organizations, recognized the major deficiencies in knowledge of health care providers. Steps were implemented including the release of national guidelines for the treatment of cancer pain and efforts to educate physicians, nurses, and other professionals to gain expertise in this critical patient care concern. A missing link to these efforts has been equal attention on the education of patients and family members as partners to improve pain control.

The *American Cancer Society's Guide to Pain Control* is an attempt to meet the challenge for better pain management. This book is a broad step forward in informing patients and their families of their right to pain relief and in describing the kind of care that patients should expect in the treatment of pain. Cancer care is a partnership of patients and professionals, and this is no truer in any aspect of oncology than the area of pain management. Effective relief of pain requires that patients communicate their pain to professionals, participate fully in using the multitude of pharmacologic therapies available, and enlist the many nondrug treatments so vital in optimum pain relief. We are extremely fortunate that there have been so many advances in the treatment of pain in recent years. There are many new medications to treat pain, ways to administer them, and key advances in controlling side effects of these treatments. Scientists have made important contributions to understanding the nature of pain and addressing specific pain problems such as nerve pain, bone pain, and pain of advanced disease.

This book should be required reading for all patients with cancer and their family members. Consumers should hold their health care providers accountable to provide the kind of pain relief that we would all seek for someone we love facing cancer. Lessons learned over the past decade of attention to this problem are clear. Patients who are newly diagnosed and beginning cancer treatment will be able to tolerate these treatments far more successfully if their pain is controlled. The ever-growing population of long-term cancer survivors cannot proceed with their lives and engage fully in their work, family, or enjoyment of other activities without ongoing relief of pain that often continues into long-term survivorship. And those who will face life's end from advanced cancer will require optimum management of pain in order to achieve quality of life at this very precious time of life. The vital message of this book is **pain can be relieved**. We have the knowledge, the medications, and the ability to relieve the vast majority of pain in people with cancer. These accomplishments will only be realized when patients and their families are supported by competent professionals who share the vision of a time when pain will not be such a feared aspect of cancer. Only then will we be able to rest confidently in the knowledge that each and every patient with cancer, young or old, will live all of the days of their lives free from pain.

Introduction

Pain is one of the most feared complications of cancer, yet many people with cancer do not have cancer-related pain. Of those who do, about nine out of ten can get effective relief. In the few situations where pain cannot be completely relieved, it can be reduced so the person with cancer can live with it and carry on most daily activities.

Today, there are many different kinds of medicines and other methods that can help relieve pain. With effective pain management, people with cancer pain can be free to sleep and eat better, enjoy the company of family and friends, and continue with work, hobbies, and other pleasurable activities.

THE IMPACT OF CANCER PAIN

In general, about two out of every three people with cancer have experienced pain sometime during their cancer experience. Although cancer pain is often thought of as a crisis that emerges in advanced stages of disease, it may occur at any stage for many reasons. The pain may be due to:

- diagnostic procedures such as a bone marrow biopsy
- surgery or other therapeutic procedures
- lymphedema
- side effects of chemotherapy and radiation
- tumor growth with compression on surrounding tissue or nerves
- limited mobility
- other illnesses or infections

The incidence of pain in patients with cancer depends on the type and stage of disease. While it is difficult to get an accurate estimate, nearly 75 percent of patients with advanced cancer have pain. Of the people with cancer who have pain, about 40 to 50 percent report it as moderate to severe, and another 25 to 30 percent describe it as very severe.

Pain can have a significant impact on both the physical and emotional aspects of life. It can cause suffering, loss of control, and impair the quality of a person's life throughout the course of care. It can reduce physical and social activity, appetite, and sleep. It can further weaken the body, and make it difficult to follow through with scheduled treatments. Uncontrolled pain prevents people from working productively, enjoying recreation, or taking pleasure in their usual roles in the family and society.

The psychological effects of cancer pain can also be devastating. A person's inability to meet financial, employment, and interpersonal demands can create a heavy burden. Mental outlook has a direct effect on how a person perceives and copes with pain. People with cancer may lose hope when pain occurs because they think pain signals the progression of disease. Chronic, severe, or unrelieved pain can lead to depression. Depression or anxiety can lower a person's tolerance for pain and make the pain feel even worse.

CANCER PAIN IS UNDERTREATED

The inadequate treatment of cancer pain causes needless suffering. Although there are a variety of treatment methods available to relieve cancer pain, research shows that it is still being undertreated. In 1990, the National Cancer Institute reported that the inadequate treatment of pain and other symptoms of cancer "is a serious and neglected public health problem."

Despite the fact that treatments exist that can significantly reduce cancer pain and improve the quality of life of patients, survivors, and their families, enormous barriers persist that prevent these treatments from being adequately and appropriately applied. Lack of knowledge on the part of patients and health professionals about the appropriate use of treatments is a major barrier. Myths and misconceptions about pain, addiction, and tolerance all contribute to reluctance by patients and health professionals to ask for and use pain medication. Health care professionals lack knowledge about how to measure and adequately treat pain. Fear of disciplinary action by licensing boards and criminal prosecution by drug enforcement agencies also inhibits professionals in actively pursuing pain control strategies with medicines.

Pain control is still considered a secondary issue, rather than a centrally important element of appropriate cancer care. Until recently, practice standards for health care systems did not include pain control. Health insurance reimbursement is lacking for pain medications, which restricts the access to needed pain control. Further, societal and cultural barriers limit patients' ease in raising concerns about cancer pain, inhibit appropriate and adequate prescription of pain medications by doctors and nurses, and deter use of these medications by patients.

METHODS OF PAIN CONTROL

Cancer pain can be treated in a variety of ways. One of the most effective methods of pain control is the use of medicines, known as drug therapy, which changes the perception of pain. Drug therapy brings significant relief in most cases. Other methods that are used to reduce the sensation of pain include nerve blocks and nervous system surgery, acupuncture, cold/heat packs, massage, transcutaneous electrical nerve stimulation (TENS), exercise, or immobilization (e.g., bracing a joint).

Pain relief can also be achieved by reducing a person's reaction to pain. People can learn skills such as relaxation, imagery, meditation, distraction, biofeedback, hypnosis, and other techniques to increase the ability to cope with pain and remain as active as possible. These complementary nondrug methods can also help people cope with the emotional and psychological impact of pain on their quality of life and well being, both of which can be significantly affected by pain.

WHAT YOU CAN DO

The first step in pain control is to identify the pain (see Chapter 3). If your doctor does not bring up the subject of pain, it is up to you to make your pain known. The cornerstone of effective pain management is a thorough pain assessment, or evaluation to determine important information about your pain. What you tell your doctor about your pain and how you describe your pain is the most important tool for measuring pain. You can help by describing your experience of pain in as much detail as possible. Only you can describe the nature of your pain to your health care team. Include the following:

- the location
- how long it lasts
- when it started
- the intensity or how severe it is
- what helps it and what makes it worse

Recording the effects of your pain and how it impacts your ability to function every day will also help with the evaluation. Your doctor will include your information along with a detailed history, physical examination, psychosocial assessment, and results of any diagnostic studies to determine the treatment options that are best for you.

WHAT THE AMERICAN CANCER SOCIETY IS DOING

The American Cancer Society (ACS) has established ambitious goals for reducing the incidence and mortality rate of cancer as well as achieving a measurable improvement in the quality of life of people with cancer and their families by the year 2015. The focus on quality of life issues is significant. Cancer mortality rates have begun to decline and the number of people living with cancer is increasing. In fact, more Americans now live with cancer, than die from the disease. Thus, the importance of quality of life issues cannot be overstated. These issues range from the physical to the spiritual and affect the person's overall perceptions of well being and survival. Pain is the one characteristic of cancer that most affects the quality of life for individuals living with the challenges of the cancer experience.

The ACS has identified pain control as one of its nationwide quality of life objectives. In August 2000, the ACS gathered a group of nationally known experts in the field of pain control and representatives from organizations involved in pain control and palliative care in order to develop a strategic plan. The specific pain control goal is to provide appropriate care for the control of pain based upon an appropriate plan of care using uniform standards for 90 percent of people with cancer by 2015. The ACS focus in addressing pain control is specific to cancer pain, and consistent with the Society's mission statement, which is dedicated to diminishing suffering from cancer through research, education, advocacy, and ensuring access to services.

Recommendations for Action

Recommendations for ACS action to reduce the burden of pain for people with cancer and their families have been developed in the following areas:

- Information About Pain Control
- Public Awareness and Education

- Patient and Family Support
- Health Care Providers
- Research
- Health Systems
- Collaboration
- Public Policy and Legislation
- Internal ACS Actions

Each target is considered an area of particular strength for the ACS, where the existing capacities and national network uniquely position the ACS to advance efforts to control pain and thereby achieve its nationwide pain control objective.

HOW TO USE THIS BOOK

The *American Cancer Society's Guide to Pain Control* is a comprehensive guide that serves as a reference for understanding all of the complex issues involved in dealing with cancer pain. The goal of this book is to provide people affected by cancer pain with the tools for:

- learning about pain
- overcoming the barriers to pain treatment
- understanding pain in order to describe it to members of the health care team
- communicating with members of the health care team
- managing pain and related side effects
- dealing with the related legal, financial, emotional, and social concerns
- finding helpful resources in your community and across the country

This book will walk you through the issues and details related to pain control from diagnosis throughout your cancer experience. You'll discover how you can get the most effective pain relief and what you can do to help yourself. As you read, you'll begin to understand how cancer pain and its treatment affect your body, your emotions, your relationships with others, and your life in general. We encourage you to evaluate the information and talk with your health care team to determine how best to treat your pain. Always remember that you have a right to receive appropriate treatment for pain control.

CHAPTER 1

Achieving Effective Pain Control

A new nurse was recently hired to work in a hospital unit with cancer patients. She admitted that she had not worked in this area before, but was willing to take the challenge. When Mrs. Allen, in Room 231, asked for pain medicine while she was laughing on the phone, the new nurse expressed her disbelief that Mrs. Allen was asking for pain medicines. "She was laughing on the phone; she wasn't having pain," was her comment. Of course, the nurses who had worked with great effort to get Mrs. Allen's severe pain under control knew that she was having pain. Thus began the long road of teaching the new nurse about oncology and the needs of people with cancer.

About two-thirds of patients currently receiving cancer treatment experience some type of pain. In most cases, cancer pain can be sufficiently controlled to allow patients to go about their daily routines, participate in important activities, and enjoy life. Although pain control is often easy to achieve, many patients who have cancer-related pain do not receive adequate care for their distress and still suffer needlessly.

There are a variety of reasons why many people with cancer do not receive adequate pain relief, ranging from poor communication between doctors and patients to irrational fears that taking pain medicine will cause patients to become addicted. Some patients may be hesitant to discuss their pain, fearing that it will cause their doctors' attention to shift away from their cancer treatment. Others may believe that expressing pain is a sign of personal weakness. Lack of knowledge among health care professionals concerning pain assessment and treatment also contributes to inadequate cancer pain management. Some doctors fear that they will encounter regulation problems if they prescribe large doses of pain medicine, even when needed by patients.

Pain can greatly lower a person's quality of life, but in most cases, it can be treated. By developing an understanding of the issues related to pain and its treatment, you can get the help you need for relieving your pain. The result will be increased well being and improved quality of life while undergoing cancer treatment and recovery.

Myths and Misconceptions About Cancer Pain

Providing knowledge and dispelling misinformation about pain and pain relief is so important that the first chapter of this book is devoted to the topic. If there were not so many barriers that stand between pain and pain relief, many people with cancer would be able to live without pain or at least live with levels of pain that do not detract significantly from their lives. The following myths and misunderstandings among both health care professionals and patients represent barriers and obstacles to effective pain treatment.

Myth #1: Pain is a normal part of having cancer. While many people with cancer experience pain, it should not be considered normal or an unavoidable consequence of having the disease. Pain is not a necessary part of cancer and it takes a major physical and emotional toll on the person experiencing the pain. Cancer itself is not a normal condition. Any pain that results from the presence of cancer should be addressed aggressively, quickly, and with all of the resources available to your health care team. When pain does occur, you can rest assured that it can be controlled in almost all circumstances.

Myth #2: Pain means that the cancer is growing. Pain is not necessarily a sign that the cancer is getting worse or is incurable, and it is not an inevitable consequence of cancer. Pain may occur at any time during the course of illness and for any number of reasons. It may even occur for people whose condition is stable and whose life expectancy is long.

Many things can cause aches and pains besides the growth of cancer. For example, patients can have headaches or backaches caused by things other than cancer.

Or they can have pain in their arm from a fall that caused a broken bone. Some pain can be caused by side effects of the cancer treatment. For example, patients who receive chemotherapy may have sores in their mouth that are very painful, or those who have radiation to the lower abdomen can have cramping with diarrhea or develop a painfully sore rectum. This pain is related to the treatment and not the cancer. People with cancer will have pain after surgery, but this does not means that the cancer is growing. It means that tissue has been cut and nerve endings have been disrupted, which causes pain. Once the nerve endings and tissue heal, the pain will go away. Sometimes cancer patients may have pain because of the location of the tumor, which will not always mean that the cancer has grown.

Myth #3: Pain can't be treated. Some people simply believe that pain is just something they have to "deal" with. They think pain is inevitable and that all they can do is accept their fate. The fact is that there are very few cases of pain that cannot be relieved. Cancer pain can almost always be relieved safely, effectively, and sometimes quickly using relatively simple methods.

Myth #4: Doctors don't understand pain. The best way for your doctor, nurse, and other treatment team members to understand your pain is to talk to them. Even if it is difficult or uncomfortable to discuss, you are the best person to explain how your pain affects your body and your life. Concerned and knowledgeable doctors and nurses can achieve good pain control for almost all of their patients, but they must be aware of your situation. You are in the best position to provide them with all of the necessary information.

Sometimes people are afraid that their health care professionals will think they are exaggerating the level of pain or are being cowardly. Some doctors and other members of the cancer care team may not be adequately trained to assess and treat cancer-related pain, or they may not understand the urgency and importance of pain relief in the larger scheme of cancer treatment. It is your right as a patient to receive assistance in pain management. In fact, if your doctor or nurse does not understand and care for your pain, seek further help from someone else.

Myth #5: Good patients don't complain. Some people don't want to be bothersome. They think they are being a burden or difficult if they talk about the pain. Some patients believe that by not "making waves" they will get more attention and better cancer treatment. Although there are effective options for controlling pain, some people endure it needlessly rather than ask their doctors to prescribe stronger or different medications or to try other treatments if the current drug therapy program is not working. People can actually be helpful to their doctors by explaining the details of their pain. This information helps doctors know the best way to treat the pain. Telling your doctor about pain will not compromise the quality of your cancer treatment.

Myth #6: Focusing on the pain may be a distraction from treating the cancer. Some patients are concerned that doctors focusing on treating their pain may do so at the risk of not treating their cancer. However, both the pain and the cancer can be treated together at the same time. In fact, the presence of pain may make it very difficult for patients to comply with cancer treatment—the very treatment that holds the promise for curing their disease and relieving their pain.

Myth #7: People should be able to "tough it out." Some people believe that they should be able to put up with the pain. Their family or cultural background may have influenced the belief that talking about pain makes a person weak (see Chapter 10). However, tolerating pain can actually make a person weak, both physically and emotionally. Unrelieved pain causes decreased appetite, disturbed sleep, diminished physical activity, and can quickly drain energy. Pain should be treated as soon as possible.

Myth #8: Pain medications lead to addiction. Probably the most widespread misconception about cancer pain treatment is that pain medications will lead to addiction, or uncontrollable drug craving, seeking, and use (see Chapter 4, pages 91–94). This unfounded worry prevents many patients from taking medications prescribed to relieve pain. The fact is that people who take cancer pain medicines, as prescribed by the doctor, rarely become addicted to them. Indeed, if the patient's pain is treated effectively, it *decreases* the risk of addiction.

If you have a history of substance abuse or other concerns about addiction, share them with those who are caring for you (see Chapter 11). These fears should not prevent you from using pain medicines to effectively relieve your pain.

Even many medical professionals, including doctors, lack thorough knowledge about pain treatment and continue to work under the impression that opioids (strong pain relievers also known as narcotics) may lead to drug addiction. Medical training often focuses on treating diseases, not on relieving symptoms. If your doctor is reluctant to prescribe pain medication when necessary, you may want to seek another opinion.

Myth #9: Taking too much pain medication over time will decrease its effectiveness. Another misconception is that your body will become immune to the effects of the pain medicine. This fear may cause you to hold off taking opioids or to save the strongest opioids for "later" when pain becomes more severe. Patients may mistakenly believe that if they save strong medications until pain becomes very bad, the drugs will be more effective. However, if you delay taking pain relief medications until your pain returns, even strong opioids will become less effective. Preventing pain and keeping it under control is easier than treating it once it becomes severe.

Some people who take opioids for pain may find that over time they need to take larger doses. This may be due to an increase in the pain or the development of drug tolerance. Drug tolerance occurs when your body gets used to the medicine you are taking, and your medicine does not relieve the pain as well as it once did. Many people do not develop a tolerance to opioids. If tolerance does develop, usually small increases in the dose or a change in the kind of medicine will help relieve the pain. Increasing the doses of opioids to relieve increasing pain or to overcome drug tolerance does *not* lead to addiction.

Myth #10: Pain medications cause unpleasant side effects. Some pain medications can cause side effects, but most diminish with time or can be managed or prevented. The potential for side effects is no reason to avoid using these highly effective pain relievers. Opioids almost always cause some degree of constipation (see Chapter 6). Drinking lots of water, eating a high-fiber diet, and using laxatives and stool softeners will counteract the constipating effects. Opioids also cause many patients to become drowsy or to fall asleep (which might actually be related to the pain having kept them from getting adequate rest). This effect usually diminishes within a few days after drug therapy begins.

Occasionally, patients become dizzy or feel confused when they take opioids. If this happens to you, tell your nurse or doctor. These side effects may disappear on their own or may be relieved by changing the dose or type of medication you take. Some people fear that opioids will make them "high" and lose control. These drugs can make you feel "spacey" and "out of it" for a short time, but your body will adjust to these changes and after a short time you will no longer notice them.

Sometimes opioids cause nausea and vomiting at first. These side effects usually disappear after a few days, or they can be managed with antinausea drugs or by changing medications or doses. If you experience side effects from your pain medicine, notify your doctor or nurse immediately so they can take steps to bring you relief.

The Importance of Communication

To receive the most effective pain treatment, you must be willing to discuss your pain clearly, accurately, honestly, and on a regular basis with members of your health care team and with caregivers at home. Everyone experiences and deals with pain differently. Even the way people talk about the type or intensity of their pain and discomfort varies, so it is important for you to describe your unique experience of pain. Many people find that talking about pain in specific terms is difficult, but the more information you can give to your doctor or nurse, the more likely a solution will be found. Telling a doctor or family member that "it hurts" is only the beginning of the description of your pain.

COMMUNICATING WITH YOUR HEALTH CARE TEAM

The first and most critical step is to make certain that your doctor, nurse, and other members of your health care team are aware of your pain and how it affects your life. Because pain is such an individual experience, you are the best judge of your pain and the consequences it has in your life. Only you know how much pain you feel, what relieves it, what makes it worse, and how your pain relief needs change over time. When discussing your pain with your health care team, be as specific as possible (see Chapter 3). Describe the pain's intensity, location, how long it lasts, how it changes, what pain relief steps work and which do not, and what psychological effects the pain creates (for example, depression, anxiety, and worry). Armed with such information, the health care professional who is in charge of your pain treatment can design a plan to meet your needs. Together, you can map out the steps you will take toward relief, including medications, nondrug therapies, or special procedures. Communicating openly and honestly with others about your cancer pain greatly increases your chances of getting the relief you need and deserve which can improve the quality of your life. Sometimes finding the right solution takes several attempts, regardless of a doctor's skill and knowledge. The process may require time and may be frustrating for patients, family, and health professionals. But, in the long run, you will be gratified that you continued to discuss your pain relief needs with your health care team.

Many concerned and compassionate health care providers are trained to focus on cancer treatment, but some simply do not realize that relieving pain is a crucial part of cancer treatment. Few medical schools include education about the importance and methods of pain relief. They typically teach students to address brief, short-lived pain (from surgery, for example), but not how to treat chronic pain that often accompanies cancer. Patients and their caregivers must make sure their doctors and nurses view pain seriously and take all necessary steps to relieve it. If necessary, insist that your pain be treated.

Cancer care is typically provided through a team approach, where the skills and talents of various medical professionals are applied to different aspects of treatment. Consider speaking with each team member about your pain and pain management needs so that you understand how each may be able to help you. When all members of the team communicate well and work together, efforts at pain relief are more likely to succeed. But do not assume that everyone on your health care team knows about your case or your pain control needs. You or a caregiver may have to make sure that all members of the health care team understand your particular experience of pain and pain relief.

Remember that you are responsible for communicating your pain control needs to your health care team. Only you know how pain affects your life and how effective various pain treatments are. Together, you and your health care team can develop an effective plan for pain relief. They need to hear about what works and what doesn't work to relieve your pain. Understanding your pain also helps them better understand how the cancer and its treatment affect your body. Discussions about pain will not distract your doctor from treating the cancer, but will result in better treatment of your disease and better symptom management. The best time to tell your doctor or nurse about pain is immediately after it begins, because pain is easier to treat when it first emerges than after it becomes troublesome or severe.

Members of Your Health Care Team

The following alphabetical list includes some of the medical professionals who are likely to help you deal with pain at different stages of your cancer treatment:

Anesthesiologist. This is a medical doctor who specializes in giving medicines or other agents that prevent or relieve pain, especially during surgery. Anesthesiologists may also work in pain clinics to treat patients with conditions that cause chronic pain.

Medical Oncologist. This is a medical doctor who sees the cancer patient once a cancer diagnosis is made. The oncologist is involved in planning the appropriate treatment for the patient and prescribes chemotherapy, hormonal therapy, and other anticancer drugs, and refers you to other specialists. He or she works with registered nurses, clinical nurse specialists, nurse practitioners, or physician assistants. Your medical oncologist may keep in contact with other members of your health care team to ensure that you receive the most effective treatment possible. He or she can keep you informed about the latest available treatments and resources.

Neurologist. This is a medical doctor who specializes in treating conditions associated with the brain, nerves, and spinal cord. Neurologists may also treat patients who suffer chronic pain.

Neurosurgeon. This is a medical doctor who specializes in surgery involving the brain, spinal cord, and nerves. To relieve pain, sometimes a neurosurgeon will conduct surgical procedures that involve cutting individual nerves, groups of nerves, or even parts of the spinal cord itself.

Nurse. During your treatment you will be in contact with different types of nurses, including registered nurses (RNs), licensed practical nurses (LPNs), and licensed vocational nurses (LVNs). RNs can monitor your condition, provide treatment, educate you about side effects, and help you adjust physically and emotionally to cancer. A *nurse practitioner* is a registered nurse with a master's or doctoral degree who can diagnose and manage cancer care. Nurse practitioners share many tasks with your doctors, such as recording your medical history, conducting physical exams, and doing follow-up care. In most states, a nurse practitioner can prescribe medications with a doctor's supervision. A *clinical nurse specialist* is a nurse who has a master's degree in a specific area, such as oncology, psychiatry, or critical care nursing. An *oncology-certified nurse* is a clinical nurse who has demonstrated an in-depth knowledge of oncology care. He or she has passed a certification exam. Oncology-certified nurses are found in all areas of oncology practice. All nurses can help to assess pain, teach patients about pain control, and monitor pain therapy programs.

Pain Specialist. This may be an oncologist, anesthesiologist, neurosurgeon, other doctor, nurse, or pharmacist. They are specially trained to relieve pain that results from many sources, including cancer. Pain specialists may be very helpful when other members of your health care team are unable to control your pain.

Personal or Primary Care Doctor. The primary care doctor has a broad, general knowledge of health care and is usually the first doctor you will meet with before being referred to proper specialists to diagnose or treat your cancer. A primary care physician may be a general practitioner, internist, family doctor, and even a medical oncologist or radiation oncologist. Your primary care doctor may or may not be involved in your cancer care. Sometimes, the primary care doctor is in charge of coordinating your care with other health care professionals and refers patients to appropriate specialists.

Pharmacist. This is an expert in how drugs affect the body and how different drugs react with one another. Doctors frequently turn to pharmacists to get information on medications. Your pharmacist is a very good source if you have questions or concerns about the medications your doctor has prescribed.

Physical Therapist/Physiotherapist. This is a specialist who has been trained to help patients return to their full function after events such as surgery or injuries that cause physical weakness or pain. The physical therapist teaches you exercises and other stretching and strengthening techniques, and also administers massage or heat to help you restore or maintain your body's strength, function, and flexibility. Physical therapists may use some massage techniques to stretch tight muscles and help relieve pain.

Physician Assistant (PA). This specialist provides health care services with supervision from physicians. PAs are formally trained to provide diagnostic, therapeutic, and preventive health care services, as delegated by a physician. Working as members of the health care team, they take medical histories, examine patients, order and interpret laboratory tests and x rays, prescribe medications (in most states), and make diagnoses.

Psychotherapist/Counselor. This specialist addresses patients' psychological well being and helps them to improve their quality of life by reducing anxiety, depression, and helplessness, all of which can accompany a cancer diagnosis. Psychotherapists can help patients develop effective coping strategies for dealing with cancer and some of its side effects such as pain and stress. They can also teach patients techniques for better communication with doctors and other members of the health care team—communication that will allow patients to more closely follow medical instructions and to ensure that their pain management needs are addressed. Therapy may be conducted individually, as well as in couples, families, and groups. Mental health professionals may include, social workers, psychologists, psychiatrists, marriage and family therapists, licensed professional counselors, pastoral counselors, and psychiatric nurses (see Chapter 7). Psychotherapists may use a number of techniques, such as relaxation, imagery, and self-hypnosis to help control pain.

Radiation Oncologist. This is a medical doctor who specializes in treating cancer with radiation (high-energy x-rays). The radiation oncologist helps you make decisions about your radiation therapy and determines what kind and how much radiation you should receive during cancer therapy. This member of your health care team evaluates you frequently during the course of treatment and at regular intervals afterward.

Social Worker. This is a health specialist who has a master's degree in social work and, in most cases, is licensed or certified by the state in which he or she works. A social worker is an expert in coordinating and providing non-medical care. He or she is trained to help you and your family deal with a range of emotional and practical problems, such as finances, child care, emotional issues, family concerns and relationships, transportation, and problems with the health care system. Social workers who are trained in cancer-related problems can counsel you about your fears, answer questions about diagnosis and treatment, and lead cancer support groups. You may meet with social workers during a hospital stay or on an outpatient basis.

Surgeon. This is a medical doctor who performs surgery. (A *surgical oncologist* specializes in using surgery to diagnose and treat cancer.) You will consult with your surgeon before and after you undergo any surgical procedure. He or she will conduct surgical diagnostic procedures to determine the location or extent of the cancer. The surgeon will then remove tumors and, if necessary, surrounding tissue. A surgeon may also operate specifically to help relieve pain. Your surgeon will work closely with surgical nurses, your anesthesiologist, and your medical oncologist and will issue a surgical report to your personal doctor and your medical oncologist that will help determine your future cancer treatment plan.

COMMUNICATING WITH CAREGIVERS

Someone, such as a family member or friend, is usually available to help and support you during your cancer treatment. These people are called caregivers. Caregivers play an important part in your pain management program (see Chapter 8). People often tolerate pain better when they get enough support from others. Caregivers can assist you by providing an outlet for discussing your pain, and by offering encouragement and emotional support. They can also help you describe your pain to health care providers, make sure that you follow your pain treatment plan, and note changes in your behavior or attitude signifying changes in your pain that should be reported to a doctor or nurse. A caregiver can also become your advocate and act as a link between you and your health care providers, and may even become an active participant in the decision-making process.

It's important that you have support from others to provide you with the reassurance and assistance you need at a time when you are struggling with pain. While you might want to be as independent as possible, dealing with pain sometimes makes that very difficult. There will be times when the help of others can make a real difference in your quality of life. Below are some tips for getting support:

- Make a list of people who can give companionship and support to you. Think about all those people that you have supported. Don't be hesitant to make an extensive list, so that you have many people from which to choose.
- Make a list of the things that need to be accomplished. It helps if you provide people with specific ways they can help. You will certainly be less stressed if some responsibilities can be shared with people who care about you.

- Access your resource network. Is there a neighbor who shops for her family every week who could call to see if you are running short on something?
- When people say to you "let me know what I can do," answer the question honestly depending on what you need. If you are vague about your needs because you're not comfortable asking for help, nothing is achieved. Speak up when someone offers help. People usually mean it when they offer to help. In fact, it gives them satisfaction to be able to do something for someone they care about.

Barriers to Communication

There are many barriers to communication that prevent patients from receiving adequate pain care. These may include language and cultural differences between patients and health care professionals, patients' inability or reluctance to discuss pain, and lack of recognition by health care workers about the importance of pain control.

LANGUAGE BARRIERS

Because pain is best reported by the person who experiences it, the ability to communicate verbally with doctors, nurses, and other health care professionals is essential to ensure that patients receive the best pain relief possible. Patients who speak a foreign language and have limited command of the English language may find it difficult to communicate with health care professionals who speak only English. They will not be able to describe their pain adequately and may not receive the appropriate amount of attention it deserves. Doctors and nurses who do not understand patients will not be able to assess their pain accurately and therefore may not be able to formulate the most effective pain management strategy.

Patients in pain may revert to their primary language because they are under stress and can't think clearly. When there is a difference in language, the medical staff may have to rely on simple visual tools to assess a patient's pain and to gauge the effects of treatment. For example, health professionals may, with the help of a translator, help a patient devise a simple, two-language verbal rating scale that both can understand and use to measure pain and pain relief.

Hospitals typically have staff members who act as translators for patients who speak foreign languages. Caregivers who understand both English and the primary language of the patient may also serve as translators. In addition, patients who do not understand English well should find out if printed instructions about cancer pain and pain control are available in languages other than English.

CULTURAL DIFFERENCES

Cultural background—which includes ethnicity, religious beliefs, personal values, morals, and family dynamics—can greatly influence how people cope with and talk about their pain. Culture influences not only how patients perceive pain, but also how and even if they are willing to discuss it with health professionals and caregivers. It affects communication styles and general attitudes about both traditional and nontraditional forms of medical care. Culture has a major impact on how individuals view pain relief measures (such as drug therapy) and how much pain they will endure before asking for help (see Chapter 10).

PAIN IS SUBJECTIVE

The subjective nature of pain can make it difficult for some people to talk about it. Each person perceives and deals with pain in a unique way. No objective test or study exists to measure how much pain a person has. Health care providers and caregivers must simply accept that patients are in as much pain as they say they are, which makes accurate assessment challenging. A level of pain that causes one person to cry out may cause another to become very quiet. People also describe their pain experiences quite differently. One might use the words "occasional" and "bearable," while another may describe the pain as "frequent" and "severe." People tend to underreport their own pain levels when meeting with doctors, often because they are more concerned about whether their cancer therapy is working. Such variations make pain assessment challenging. Determining how much pain a person is in provides doctors with an important baseline from which to develop pain management strategies.

If you are in pain, you need to be able to describe it to your doctor and other members of your health care team (see Chapter 3). This can be difficult for some people, who find it hard to talk about their pain in detailed terms. Try to use

Tips for Communicating
with Doctors and Caregivers

- Tell your doctors and caregivers about any concerns you may have so they can help find a solution.
- If you don't understand something, ask that it be repeated, rephrased, or explained clearly. You might say, "I'm having trouble grasping what you said, would you mind telling me again," or "could you put it another way?" Another tactic is to repeat what was said and ask for confirmation, "Let me see if I have it right. You're saying that…"
- Prepare a list of questions ahead of time. Ask the most important ones first and ask as many as you need.
- Make sure that all your concerns and questions have been addressed by your doctor or nurse, no matter how small they seem. It may take more than one visit to discuss all of your concerns, because new questions may come to mind after you return home.
- Be direct with others and express your needs and feelings.
- If you and your family usually don't talk about certain personal issues, it's okay not to completely open up to everyone.
- Speak out if someone offends you. When people are being insensitive, let them know.
- Learn as much as possible about what is happening and what may happen in the future. This can reduce fears of the unknown.
- Explain your thoughts and fears to an understanding person, whether a

words that will help others understand what you feel. Pain has different effects on different people. Don't hesitate to talk about your pain to those who can help you. A pain management plan cannot be effective if you fail to report pain. You have a right to the best pain control you can get. Relieving your pain means you can continue to do the everyday things that are important to you. Remember, only you know what you are feeling.

LIMITED KNOWLEDGE AND TIME

Poor communication may result when health care providers are inadequately trained to assess pain properly and are not familiar with the most current pain friend or therapist. Talking to understanding people will show you that others empathize with you and can help you think through the impact of your emotions.

- Express your emotions as you wish, although you may feel that you don't want to share your emotions and feelings with everyone. It's okay to be alone, but be aware that there are people with whom you can talk.
- Sharing doesn't always mean talking. You may feel more comfortable writing about your feelings.
- Having a sense of control over what happens to you makes a difficult experience easier to manage. Gathering information about your pain, participating in treatment decisions, and knowing what to expect can counteract feelings that your situation is hopeless. It is not necessary to learn every detail, ask every question, and make all the decisions. You can gain control by making sure you have a health care team that you trust to recommend and provide the best care you need.
- Pain is in *your* body and is affecting *your* life. Therefore, it's up to you to determine your priorities and needs. Trust your doctors and listen carefully to what they say. But before you decide on a treatment program, make sure you're informed enough to feel confident that the treatment plan you and your doctor have structured is what's best for you. Explore and clarify every aspect of treatment before beginning.

management strategies. Some simply may not realize the tremendous impact pain has on a person's life. Others may not communicate clearly to patients the importance of closely following their pain treatment plans. These days, many doctors are under great pressure to keep visits short and are so preoccupied with cancer treatment that they don't pay adequate attention to a patient's pain. They may not understand that a patient in pain is less likely to comply with important cancer treatment instructions. Some doctors inaccurately judge a patient's severity of pain and minimize the importance of pain and pain treatment. Your pain may slip by unnoticed if you don't speak up.

When to Seek Additional Help

You should expect your doctor to take all the necessary steps to relieve your pain and make you as comfortable as possible. But when pain relief strategies prescribed by your doctor do not succeed, it may be time to seek help elsewhere.

Talk frankly with your doctor and make it clear that you require better pain relief and more attention paid to your pain. Ask to be referred to a pain specialist or a pain clinic. New developments in pain management occur regularly, and your doctor may simply not be familiar with all of them. A doctor who has your best interest at heart and has genuinely tried to help relieve your pain in a sensitive and caring manner should not hesitate to help you find other sources of pain control. However, if you are in pain and your doctor doesn't seem to take your situation seriously or does not offer alternatives, seek treatment elsewhere.

Pain programs or specialists can be located through a cancer center, a hospice, or the oncology department at a local hospital or medical center. The American Cancer Society and other organizations may also be able to provide information on pain specialists, pain clinics, or programs in your area. It is your right to seek appropriate care to relieve pain, and ultimately it is up to you to ensure that you get the care you need and deserve.

CHAPTER 2

Understanding Cancer Pain

After she was first diagnosed, Melissa was afraid that she would have pain. Actually, she thought cancer and pain went hand in hand. She had pain with her surgery, but it was well controlled and soon went away. After surgery, she feared having more pain even though her cancer had been removed. She could not block the memories of her father dying in pain from his cancer. She expected to have pain just like him. But, she has been without any evidence of disease for nine years. And no pain.

One of the first steps in managing your pain is learning about your pain. Although you may be afraid of pain, you should know that having cancer does not always mean having pain. If pain does occur, there are many ways to relieve or reduce it. This chapter will discuss the nature of pain and give you the language needed to help you talk with your health care team about your pain.

What Is Pain?

Pain is a sensation that hurts. It is a warning signal that something is wrong in our bodies. It can have many causes in people with cancer, however, not all people with cancer will experience pain. Physically, pain can range from mildly discomforting to severely agonizing or debilitating. Not only do people's perceptions of pain differ, but their reactions to pain are different. Some people experience pain for only a short period of time, while others may have to deal with chronic pain for months, seriously impacting the quality of their lives.

Pain has two main components: a sensory component and a reactive component. The sensory component involves the transmission, or sending of, the pain signal from the injured part of the body to the spinal cord and brain. When the pain signal is received, the brain then sends a message to the person that he or she is having pain. The reactive component refers to how the person reacts to the pain. This reaction depends on the person's pain threshold (the intensity of the stimulus a person considers painful) and his or her pain tolerance (how intense or how long the pain stimulus can persist before the person experiences the pain). People can have differences in their pain thresholds and pain tolerances.

Types of Pain

People with pain have different types of pain depending on the source of their pain. Cancer pain can result from three main causes. Most cancer pain is caused by the cancer itself. It can also occur because of the side effects of cancer treatment such as radiation therapy, chemotherapy, and surgery, and from causes not related to the cancer.

Pain can be grouped as acute, chronic, or breakthrough depending on how long the pain is present and when it occurs. It can also be categorized as nociceptive or neuropathic pain according to the words people use to describe the sensation of pain (see Chapter 3). These terms sometimes suggest the cause of the pain.

ACUTE PAIN

Acute pain is usually severe, begins suddenly, and lasts a relatively short time. It is usually a signal that body tissue is being injured in some way, and the pain generally disappears when the injury heals. An increase in blood pressure and a rapid heartbeat may also occur. Acute pain is experienced when someone has surgery, a burn, a cut, or a needle stick. Some forms of cancer treatment can also lead to acute pain such as sores in the mouth from chemotherapy, inflammation of the rectal area after radiation treatment for prostate cancer, or surgery to remove a tumor. Acute pain is usually detected more easily because of the severity of the symptoms. Acute pain that lasts for more than a few weeks becomes chronic pain.

CHRONIC PAIN

Chronic pain, which can range from mild to severe, may be ongoing and last for several months. It can result from the cancer itself or from treatment. For example the most common type of pain in people with cancer is bone pain caused by the cancer spreading to the bone. Pain caused by a tumor pressing on organs or nerves is another type of chronic pain. After the chronic pain has been present for a while, the body will adjust to this type of pain and the physical intensity will be lessened, but the impact on quality of life can still be severe. Having to deal with chronic pain on a daily basis can lead to irritability, disturbed sleep, reduced appetite, difficulty concentrating, and changes in mood, personality, lifestyle, and ability to function. Because dealing with chronic pain can make even the simplest tasks and daily activities impossible, feelings of hopelessness and depression can easily occur. These kinds of negative thoughts and emotions can make pain feel worse. To reduce this overall suffering, pain should be treated as quickly as possible.

BREAKTHROUGH PAIN

Many people with chronic cancer pain have two types of pain: persistent (continuous) pain and breakthrough (incident) pain. Persistent pain is present for long periods of time, in most cases, all day long. Breakthrough pain is a brief and often severe flare of pain that occurs even though a person may be taking pain medicine regularly for persistent pain. It's called breakthrough pain because it is pain that "breaks through" a regular pain medicine schedule.

Breakthrough pain may be different for each person and is often unpredictable. It typically comes on quickly, lasts only a few minutes or as long as an hour, and feels much like persistent pain except that it is more severe. It is common for people with persistent pain to experience episodes of breakthrough pain as well. Breakthrough pain usually has the same cause as persistent pain. It may be caused by the cancer itself or it may be related to the treatment of cancer. For some people, breakthrough pain occurs when they do a certain activity, like walking or dressing. For others, it occurs unexpectedly without any clear cause.

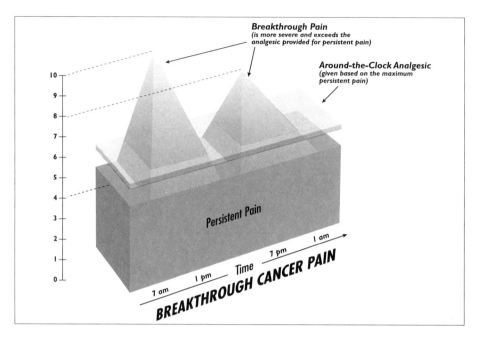

In this example, the individual has a persistent or usual pain of "4" and is taking an around-the-clock analgesic, such as a long-acting opioid (narcotic) to treat the pain. However, this patient also has two episodes of breakthrough pain: a pain of "10" at 1 P.M. and a pain of "8" at 7 P.M. He will need a medication to use for the breakthrough pain that acts quickly to relieve this pain.

NOCICEPTIVE PAIN

Nociceptive pain involves damage to body tissue. When an injury to the body occurs, pain receptors (thousands of nerve endings located throughout the body called nociceptors) are activated, sending a signal to the spinal cord and brain. This sensory information is then interpreted as pain. Nociceptors are usually turned off and only send pain signals once the body is injured or perceived to be in danger. When cancer spreads to muscle, bone, organs, and joints, the resulting pain is called nociceptive pain. Nociceptive pain is easier to locate than neuropathic pain.

NEUROPATHIC PAIN

Neuropathic pain is caused by injury to, or compression of, the structures of the nervous system which include the peripheral nerves and the central nervous system. It can result from either the cancer itself or from treatment. People often describe neuropathic pain as severe burning, sharp, tingling, or shooting. It can also cause a loss of feeling in a specific area or a feeling of extreme tenderness, making the lightest touch painful.

An example of neuropathic pain is the post-mastectomy syndrome. Following surgery, a person may experience postoperative pain but may recover from the pain and return to normal activities. Sometime later, pain may return to the same area with no cause of the pain being found. The pain may be described as "weird" or "strange," and burning, pressure, shooting, stabbing, or knife-like sensations. There may be pain or numbness. This is referred to as a post-mastectomy syndrome with pain resulting from damage to the nerves in that area of the body.

Factors That Intensify Pain

Pain thresholds and pain tolerances differ from person to person, but how pain is perceived depends on how it is processed by someone's feelings, thoughts, and memories of pain. Past experiences with pain or the meaning of the pain can influence a person's reaction to a new pain. For example, people who have seen the death of a friend or family member who was in pain may be terrified at the thought of pain because they associate pain with death. However, for a professional baseball pitcher, pain resulting from a sprained ankle may be perceived quite differently (perhaps minimized or ignored) because his life is not in danger and he is receiving significant reward for ignoring the pain and continuing to play.

Some people feel hopeless or helpless in the presence of pain. Others feel alone, embarrassed, inadequate, angry, frightened, or frantic. These strong emotions can have a significant effect on how people experience pain and how they deal with it. Research has shown that the mind has a strong connection to the body, which can be either positive or negative.

Factors such as rest, understanding, support, use of analgesics, and reduction in anxiety can raise the pain threshold. However, other factors such as fatigue, depression, or anxiety can lower the pain threshold and make the pain feel worse. Fatigue is usually the result of cancer treatment. Depression and anxiety are usually the result of how a person is reacting to pain or the fear of cancer itself (see Chapter 8). Dealing with these factors, and their underlying causes, is important to reduce pain and the reaction to pain.

FATIGUE

Fatigue is the term used when a person has less energy to do the things one normally does, or wants to do. The fatigue experienced by a person with cancer is different from the normal fatigue of everyday life. It is one of the most common side effects of cancer treatment and can last from weeks to several months after treatment ends. Weakness and fatigue can also be the result of advanced cancer, depression, or medicine side effects.

Cancer-related fatigue can affect many aspects of a person's life. For example, fatigue may make it difficult to continue normal activities or enjoyable things, such as the outdoors, shopping, or dining out. Fatigue also makes it more difficult to deal with pain. And, the more tired a person becomes, the worse the pain may feel. Having to deal with fatigue can lead to depression and anxiety because the person feels helpless to change the situation—all of which may intensify pain.

Because fatigue can impact life in many ways, it should be dealt with as early as possible. Anyone with fatigue should discuss it with members of the health care team. Early treatment can help reduce the fatigue. The health care team may recommend some supportive therapies such as yoga, meditation, or music therapy as part of the treatment plan (see Chapter 7).

Causes of Pain

DIAGNOSTIC PROCEDURES

In order to make an accurate cancer diagnosis and to determine the extent of the illness, some diagnostic procedures are necessary. Some of these procedures may cause temporary pain and discomfort, lasting only for the duration of the test or a day or two afterwards. More invasive procedures may have pain that lasts several days or longer. The following are some of the most common diagnostic procedures that can cause pain or discomfort.

About Fatigue

What to Look For:
- Having no energy
- Sleeping more
- Not wanting to do normal activities
- Decreased attention to personal appearance
- Feeling tired even after sleeping
- Having trouble concentrating

What to Do:
- Plan rest periods to conserve energy for important things
- Schedule necessary activities throughout the day rather than all at once; light activity or exercise may be helpful
- Get enough rest and sleep
- Eat a nutritious diet and drink plenty of liquids
- Let others help you with meals, housework, or errands

Do Not:
- Force yourself to do more than you can manage
- Think that you are just being "lazy"

Call the Doctor:
- If you are too tired to get out of bed for more than a 24-hour period
- If you become confused
- If the fatigue becomes progressively worse
- If you have severe or frequent dizziness
- If you feel out of breath

Biopsy

A biopsy is the removal of a sample of tissue to see whether cancer cells are present. Biopsies are done with some type of device, often a sterile knife or needle, to remove the tissue. Some biopsies can be done on an outpatient basis while others may require a hospital stay. A needle biopsy may cause discomfort and pain at the site of insertion but it is temporary. A more invasive procedure such as a surgical biopsy may involve postoperative pain and discomfort.

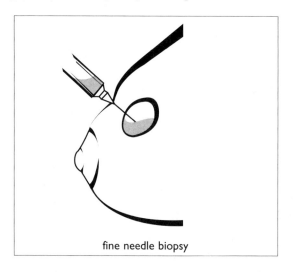

fine needle biopsy

Bone Marrow Aspiration and Biopsy

A bone marrow aspiration involves removing a small amount of bone marrow, the soft material inside bones where blood cells are formed. During a biopsy, a small cylindrical piece of bone and bone marrow (about 1/16-inch in diameter and 1/2-inch long) is removed. A local anesthetic is applied before the needle is inserted into the skin. Often, a sharp jolt and a sensation of intense pressure can be felt when the marrow is withdrawn. The puncture site may also be bruised and tender for a few days.

Endoscopy

This is a medical procedure for viewing the interior of the body through a hollow, tube-like instrument. An endoscopy may be advised if the tumor is located in an internal organ. There are many different kinds of endoscopes (the instruments used for this procedure). Each type is specially designed for examining a different part of the body, such as the stomach or colon.

Some endoscopes not only allow the doctor to see inside the body, but they can also be used for surgery. Small instruments operated through the hollow endoscope are used to remove biopsy specimens (small pieces of tissue used for laboratory tests). Biopsy samples are often taken from abnormal-appearing

Endoscopes and Body Areas Examined

You can identify these instruments because their names usually end in the suffix "scope." Of course, some instruments ending in "scope" (such as a telescope, microscope, periscope, etc.) are not endoscopes. Some types of endoscopes and the areas of the body they are used to examine are listed below:

Type of Endoscope	Body Area(s) Examined
Bronchoscope	Bronchus (breathing tubes of lungs)
Colposcope	Cervix and vagina
Cystoscope	Urinary bladder
Esophagogastroduodenoscope	Esophagus (swallowing tube) Stomach Duodenum (first part of small intestine)
Hysteroscope	Inside of uterus
Laparoscope	Cavity of abdomen and pelvis
Proctosigmoidoscope	Rectum and sigmoid colon (lower parts of large intestine)
Thorascope	Cavity of thorax (chest)

growths through an endoscope to find out if they are cancerous. A small brush can be operated through an endoscope to sample cells from the surface of a growth. Cells picked up by the brush are then used for cytology (another lab test for cancer). Sometimes an entire growth can be removed through an endoscope, or a laser beam can be operated through the endoscope to vaporize a growth.

Sometimes, endoscopy can be used instead of an actual surgical operation to get a biopsy sample or even remove or destroy a tumor. In other cases, endoscopy is used to look at a tumor and take a biopsy sample in order to decide if an actual surgical operation is needed.

There have been many advances in endoscopy during the past few years. More endoscopes are using fiberoptics (tiny fibers or wires that carry light). Fiberoptic endoscopes allow the doctor to see around corners. This can be very important in examining organs like the intestines that bend at several points. Many endoscopes are now attached to video cameras that allow doctors to view the inside of the body more clearly on a television-like screen. Also, there have been many recent advances in making surgical instruments smaller and smaller so that they can be used through an endoscope.

Because there is sometimes discomfort during an endoscopy, anesthesia or sedatives may be used. The procedure can be performed on an outpatient basis, in a doctor's office, or it may require a hospital stay. The recovery time varies depending upon the method used.

TYPES OF ENDOSCOPY

Bronchoscopy. In a bronchoscopy, a lighted, flexible tube is passed through the mouth into the bronchi of the lungs. This test can help find tumors or it can be used to take samples of tissue or fluids. This procedure may cause some throat irritation or coughing. Intravenous lines are used so medicine can be given through a vein. Medicine may be given before the test to help the person relax, but stay awake for the test.

Sigmoidoscopy. This test allows a doctor to look inside the sigmoid colon (the lower part of the large intestine or colon) and the rectum. A sigmoidoscope, a slender, flexible, hollow, lighted tube will be used to do the test. This allows the doctor to look for bleeding, cancer, and polyps. Polyps are small growths that can become cancerous. A sigmoidoscopy may be somewhat uncomfortable, but it should not be painful. The procedure takes ten to twenty minutes. Bleeding and puncture of the colon are rare complications of sigmoidoscopy.

The sigmoidoscope is lubricated so it is easy to insert into the rectum, although it may feel cool. The test is performed while the person is awake, but medicine may be given before the test to help with relaxation. To ease discomfort and the urge to have a bowel movement, it is helpful to breathe deeply but slowly through the mouth. The sigmoidoscope may stretch the wall of the colon so it feels like muscle spasms or lower abdominal pain. Air will be placed into the sigmoid colon through the sigmoidoscope so the doctor can see the colon better. During the procedure, there is a feeling of pressure and slight cramping in the lower abdomen because the air can cause gas-like pain. This slight discomfort disappears afterwards when the air leaves the colon.

Colonoscopy. This is a test used to view the lining of the colon with a colonoscope, a slender, flexible, hollow lighted tube about the thickness of a finger. It is inserted through the rectum up into the colon. A colonoscopy usually does not cause pain, although it may be uncomfortable because of the air that is injected into the bowel. The colonoscope will deliver air into the colon so that it is easier to see the lining of the colon and use the instruments to perform the test. The person may feel an urge to have a bowel movement when the colonoscope is inserted or pushed further up the colon. A polyp can be removed or a biopsy can be done during the procedure.

A colonoscopy usually lasts thirty to sixty minutes. Intravenous lines are used so medicine can be given through a vein. The test is performed while the person is awake, but medicine may be given before the test to help with relaxation. Bleeding and puncture of the colon are rare complications of colonoscopy.

Mediastinoscopy. This procedure involves the removal of tissue samples from the lymph nodes along the windpipe through a small hole cut into the neck. A mediastinoscopy involves surgery and general anesthesia (while the patient is asleep). There may be pain at the incision site.

Endometrial Biopsy

An endometrial biopsy is an office procedure in which a sample of endometrial tissue is removed by a small biopsy instrument inserted into the uterus through the cervix. The discomfort is similar to severe menstrual cramps and can be helped by taking a nonsteroidal anti-inflammatory drug such as ibuprofen an hour before the procedure. Endometrial tissue sampling can be uncomfortable and some cramping may be experienced. However, the degree and duration of pain vary.

Lumbar Puncture (Spinal Tap)

A lumbar puncture is a test in which a needle is placed in the lower back into the spinal canal to obtain a small sample of cerebrospinal fluid. This fluid is examined under a microscope to see if cancer cells are present. A painful and severe headache can develop after undergoing this procedure. The pain, which feels worse when standing up, can last from a few hours to several days. The headache can usually be treated with bed rest and medication.

There are many different ways to treat cancer, but the main types of treatment are surgery, chemotherapy, and radiation. Because each treatment is different and the treatment selected for each person will depend on the person's overall health, kind of cancer, and stage of the disease, it is difficult to predict who will experience pain from a particular treatment.

As much fear as pain instills in people, there is no need to suffer through pain without some kind of help. Learning to talk to the doctor, nurse, or someone on the health care team about pain can bring the relief that most people with cancer-related pain need and deserve. Living with pain does not need to be a standard part of the cancer treatment.

Surgery

Surgery is the oldest form of treatment for cancer. Today, surgery offers the greatest chance for cure for many types of cancer. About 60 percent of people with cancer will have some type of surgery. The pain experienced by people after surgery is generally of two types:

- Acute, short-term (temporary) pain—focused around the area of incision (surgical cutting), which is related to the healing and recovery process.
- Chronic or long-term pain—resulting from trauma (injury) to nerves, muscles, organs, or other tissue in the area where cancerous tumors and other tissue may have been removed.

Most surgical procedures to remove a tumor and surrounding tissue will require a period of recovery. During this period, it is normal for some people to feel worse than they did before the operation. After surgery, the person may feel tired, sore, and generally uncomfortable until the surgical incision is fully healed and moving about is easier. Other pain-related problems may include difficulty urinating or gas pain if there has been surgery to the abdominal area. Pain during intercourse is also very common after vaginal surgery for some gynecologic cancers. The pain associated with these procedures is common after surgery and will go away after several days. During this time, the pain can be controlled. Good pain control promotes a speedier recovery because it allows a person to be more mobile after surgery enabling him or her to leave the hospital sooner.

Some people may experience chronic pain resulting from damage to the body or nerves during surgery. Pain resulting from nerve damage is much more difficult to treat. Surgery can also result in some painful side effects such as lymphedema or phantom limb pain, both of which can occur after the removal of an appendage or body part.

Nerve Pain from Surgical Procedures

Some surgical procedures can cause injury to underlying nerves, which can lead to chronic pain for some people. This kind of pain can develop weeks or months after surgery and is usually located at the incision site. The most common surgical procedures that can lead to nerve pain are listed in the table on page 36.

Lymphedema

Mastectomy, or removal of the breast, can include removal of lymph nodes and vessels under the arm. When the lymph nodes are removed, a painful side effect known as lymphedema can occur. Lymphedema can cause painful swelling in the arm, which can range from mild to severe. This side effect can develop soon after surgery or many months or even years later. One of the first symptoms of lymphedema might be a slight feeling of tightness around the arm or hand on the side of the body treated for breast cancer.

Lymphedema affects about one in five women who have had some of their lymph nodes removed. The removal of lymph nodes and vessels changes the way the lymph fluid flows within that side of the upper body, making it more difficult for fluid in the arm to leave that area. If the remaining lymph vessels cannot remove enough of the fluid in the breast and underarm area, the excess fluid builds up and causes swelling, or lymphedema. Lymphedema usually develops slowly over time. Women undergoing any type of surgery for breast cancer should talk to someone on their health care team about the possibility of developing lymphedema.

Phantom Limb Pain

When a body part is removed during surgery, such as in a mastectomy or amputation, the person may still feel pain or other unpleasant sensations as if they were coming from the absent limb or breast. When this occurs with a limb removal, the pain is called phantom limb pain. This pain is not only physically

Surgical Procedures
Most Likely to Lead to Nerve Pain

Surgical Procedure

Mastectomy

In a simple (total) mastectomy, the surgeon removes the entire breast, but does not cut away any lymph nodes from under the arm, or muscle tissue from beneath the breast. In a modified radical mastectomy, the surgeon removes the entire breast and some of the axillary (underarm) lymph nodes. This is the most common surgery for women with breast cancer in whom the whole breast is removed. Radical mastectomy is an extensive operation removing the entire breast, axillary lymph nodes, and the pectoral (chest wall) muscles under the breast.

Radical Nephrectomy

A radical nephrectomy removes the whole kidney, the attached adrenal gland, and the fatty tissue immediately around the kidney.

Radical Neck Dissection

When certain types of cancer spread to the lymph nodes, a neck dissection is sometimes performed. There are many types of neck dissections. A radical neck dissection removes nearly all lymph nodes on one side of the neck as well as some muscles, nerves, and veins.

Thoracotomy

Surgery to the chest to remove or diagnose tumors in the lung. The surgeon must cut through ribs to get to the lungs.

uncomfortable, but it can cause emotional anxiety as well. Although medical experts are not sure why it occurs, this type of pain is very real and should be treated.

Phantom limb pain can appear months or years after surgery and may involve stump pain at the area of amputation or scar, or a burning sensation that may feel worse during movement. Some people may feel reluctant to talk about this type of

Burning, tightness, or squeezing sensations in the arm, axilla, and anterior chest wall. Pain may be worse when the arm is moved.

Heavy or bloated sensations, or numbness in the side, front part of the abdomen, and groin. Dysesthesias (sensations of pricks by pins and needles) are common.

After surgery, a tight, burning sensation may be present in the neck area. Other common side effects include numbness of the ear, weakness in raising the arm above the head, and weakness of the lower lip. These weaknesses may be permanent.

Cut ribs will hurt for a few weeks after surgery and there will be some limitations to strenuous activity. The surgical scar may feel tender and sore, or there may be a loss of feeling at the site.

pain. Obviously, it seems strange to have pain in a part of the body that no longer exists. However, this pain can be effectively treated if the health care team is aware of the pain. No single pain relief method will control phantom limb pain in all patients all the time; however, a variety of treatments may be used including pain medication, physical therapy, and nerve stimulation (see Chapters 4 and 5).

Chemotherapy

Chemotherapy is the use of anticancer medicines to kill cancer cells. They enter the bloodstream and reach all parts of the body. Chemotherapy may be used along with surgery and other types of treatment in hopes of a cure, or as a means of relieving symptoms in advanced cancer. There are people who take chemotherapy and experience no painful side effects at all; however, this is not always the case.

If the chemotherapy is given by needle in the vein, some people experience mild pain from the constant use of needles, especially when several cycles of chemotherapy are involved over several months time. However, there are devices available that can help minimize the number of times needles have to be used to deliver the drugs used in chemotherapy.

One of the most common and painful side effects of chemotherapy is stomatitis (mouth or throat sores). Similar changes in the throat or the esophagus (the tube that leads from the throat to the stomach) are called pharyngitis and esophagitis. The term mucositis is used to refer to inflammation of the lining layer of the mouth, throat, and esophagus. Certain chemotherapy drugs can cause the mouth, gums, and throat to feel sore and become red and inflamed. The tongue may also become "coated" and swollen, leading to difficulty swallowing, eating, and talking. Stomatitis, pharyngitis, and esophagitis can lead to bleeding, painful ulceration, and infection. These conditions make it difficult to eat or drink, especially when they are severe, which can lead to poor nutrition in some cases. It is important to treat mouth and throat sores quickly to reduce their impact on the person with cancer. They are most often treated with pain medication and topical anesthetics (numbing medication) which can be applied directly to the sores.

Some chemotherapy drugs irritate all mucous membranes in the body. This includes the lining of the vagina, which often becomes dry and inflamed, sometimes leading to pain during intercourse.

During chemotherapy administration into a vein, there is the possibility of extravasation (a drug leaking out of the vein). When some chemotherapy medicines are given, extravasation can lead to damage of the tissue in the area where the medicine leaks out of the vein. The pain from tissue damage can range from mild to severe, sometimes requiring plastic surgery in serious cases. However, the possibility of extravasation is decreased when a highly skilled medical professional administers the medication.

One possible side effect of some chemotherapy medicines is peripheral neuropathy, or nerve damage in which the nerves that send sensations from the hands, fingers, feet, and toes are damaged. This can lead to pain, tingling sensations, numbness, and sometimes loss of function in hands, fingers, feet, and toes.

When steroids are given as part of cancer treatment, they can cause bones to weaken (osteoporosis). Bone destruction can occur over time, which can cause chronic bone pain.

Radiation Therapy

Radiation therapy is another commonly used treatment for cancer. Advances in technology and a better understanding of how radiation works in the body have made radiation therapy a significant part of cancer treatment. It is estimated that from 50 to 60 percent of all people with cancer will receive radiation at some point during their cancer treatment.

Radiation therapy (or radiotherapy) uses an invisible ray or beam, which is focused on a region of the body where the cancer is located. In some situations, a small pellet containing a radioactive substance may be put into the tumor. Radiation can decrease the size of tumors and relieve symptoms. Some cancers can be cured by radiation therapy (Hodgkin's disease, for instance), and other cancers (breast cancers, for example) can now be treated more effectively by radiation and more limited surgical procedures.

Some of the side effects of radiation treatment can cause pain and discomfort. For example, skin exposed to radiation treatment may burn, peel, or develop sores. Sores can be quite painful and can put a person at risk for infection. Appropriate skin care measures are used to minimize these skin effects. Radiation therapy can cause damage to any tissue in the field of the radiation. This can include bones, nerves, and organs. Damage to these parts can result in pain. If the spinal cord is in the radiation field, pain will occur in various parts of the body depending on the level of damage.

The mucous membranes, as in the lining of the mouth, are also sensitive to radiation. Some mouth cancers may require high doses of radiation. A dry mouth, change in taste and mucositis (inflammation of the lining of the mouth) may occur with radiation to the head and neck area. Keeping the oral cavity clean is important to reduce the chance of infection. It may be difficult to eat if the mouth becomes tender and painful. Pain medications or topical anesthetics (medication to numb the mouth) before meals may make it easier to eat. If the pain and irritation become too severe, some people may need to have a feeding tube inserted into their stomach for nutrition.

Pelvic Radiation Therapy. For women undergoing radiation treatment to the pelvic area, pain may be associated with pink and inflamed vaginal tissue, somewhat like a sunburn. The vaginal pain and tenderness may last for a few weeks after the radiation is stopped. A few women get ulcers, or sore spots, in their vaginas. It may take several weeks or even months (in some cases) after the end of radiation therapy for these areas to heal.

Other pain stemming from radiation therapy includes pain during intercourse due to changes in the size and moistness of the vagina. Sometimes the pain sets off a problem called vaginismus. If a woman has vaginismus, the muscles around the opening of the vagina become tense. Her partner's penis cannot enter the vagina. If he pushes harder, the woman's pain is greater since her vaginal muscles are clenched in a spasm.

Radiation therapy to the male genital area can cause temporary pain during ejaculation, decreased semen volume, and genital skin irritation.

TUMOR-RELATED PAIN

Tumor-related pain can affect many different parts of the body. The type and degree of pain will vary with size and location of the tumor.

Gastrointestinal (GI) Obstruction

Pain in the abdomen can be the result of blockage (obstruction) of the stomach, small intestines, or colon. This can cause diarrhea, constipation, abdominal swelling, cramping, nausea, or vomiting. This sometimes occurs with colorectal or ovarian cancer; however, GI obstruction can also occur from any tumor that begins in or spreads to the abdomen.

Different types of abdominal pain can occur with tumors in different parts of the abdomen. For example, a tumor in the liver can cause a dull constant pain and feeling of fullness; one in the pancreas can cause mid-stomach aching pain that spreads to the middle of the back and is aggravated by lying flat; and stomach involvement is a burning pain like an ulcer or dull constant pain. A tumor in the pelvic region may be caused by bowel, ovarian, or uterine cancer. It is

Pain-Related Side Effects of Radiation

Radiation Site	Pain-Related Side Effect
Lower abdomen	Proctitis (irritation of the rectum), vaginitis (irritation of the vagina), cramping with diarrhea
Chest	Sore throat, pain with cough or deep breath, heartburn, skin irritation
Head and neck	Sore throat, esophagitis (irritation of the esophagus), skin irritation

vague and hard to pinpoint but feels full, pressure, or discomfort on both sides of the body, may be intermittent and shooting, or feel like a red-hot poker.

Intracranial Pressure/Metastases of the Skull

Tumors within any part of the brain may cause increased pressure within the skull, sometimes referred to as intracranial pressure. Increased pressure within the skull may cause headaches, nausea, vomiting, or blurred vision. More than half of people with brain tumors experience headaches involving steady, aching, dull pain. Strenuous coughing can make the headache seem worse and pain may be increased in the morning. Cancer that has spread to the base of the skull (metastases) may cause face, neck, or shoulder pain, headaches, or pain when moving the head. Head and neck pain can be a sign of spinal cord compression from a tumor.

Spinal cord compression is one of the most serious complications of bone metastasis. In this condition, pressure on the spinal cord caused by metastases extending from the spinal bones or by collapse of the spinal bones can cause pain, numbness, or paralysis. Spinal cord compression can also occur when other cancers spread to the spine as in prostate cancer.

Bone Pain

Bone metastasis (cancer that has spread to the bone) is one of the most frequent causes of pain in people with cancer and can also cause fractures, hypercalcemia (high blood calcium levels due to release of calcium from damaged bones), spinal cord compression, as well as other symptoms and complications that negatively affect a person's quality of life. Breast, prostate, kidney, lung, pancreatic, colorectal, stomach, thyroid, and ovarian cancers account for most metastases to bones. The spine is the area most often affected by bone metastasis, followed by the pelvis, hip, and upper leg bones, and the skull.

Bone pain is often the earliest sign of bone metastasis, but it is not always the only symptom. The pain often comes and goes at first, tends to be worse at night, and may be relieved by movement. Later on, it becomes a constant dull ache and may be worse during activity. Fractures (broken bones) due to bone metastasis can cause severe pain and, because they heal slowly if at all, can severely limit mobility. One of the most common symptoms of multiple myeloma, a type of cancer formed by malignant plasma cells, is bone pain. This can cause small areas of bone weakness that are often painful and osteoporosis (widespread bone weakness). Any bone may be affected, but pain over the backbone, hipbones, and skull are particularly common.

Nerve Pain

Nerve damage can cause disturbing and sometimes debilitating pain. It causes sensations such as tingling, burning, pressing, squeezing, pinching, itching, and numbness. Nerve pain is usually constant and steady and is sometimes accompanied by shooting or jolting pain, similar to a seizure or convulsion.

Nerve damage can be accompanied by bladder or bowel weakness, motor or reflex problems, or impaired senses such as poor taste or smell. Some patients also suffer from what is known as evoked pain, an unpleasant abnormal sensation in which a patient exhibits unusual pain sensitivity from something as ordinary as touch.

PAIN CAUSED BY OTHER ILLNESSES

Having cancer does not make a person immune to other illnesses. Pain can occur by illnesses not related to the cancer. Some of the more common reasons for pain include stomach problems, back strain, migraine headaches, shingles (herpes zoster), arthritis, inflammation and infection, and injuries.

Pain from stiffness can occur when a person undergoing cancer treatment is too fatigued to exercise or move around normally. Difficulty in moving is a problem characterized by general weakness and problems with walking. When a person spends a lot of time in bed, the muscles tend to weaken. It is important to move and exercise as much as possible to prevent problems associated with immobility, such as poor or no appetite, constipation, skin sores, problems with breathing, stiff joints, and mental changes.

Constipation is the infrequent or difficult passage of hard feces (stool), which often causes pain and discomfort. It is caused by too little fluid or not enough movement in the bowel. Lack of activity, general weakness, avoiding the urge to have bowel movement, pain medications, and decreased fluid intake can each contribute to this problem (see Chapter 6).

A skin or pressure sore (bedsore) can develop when the blood flow to an area of the body is reduced and the skin in that area dies. A person who is bedridden or always in a wheelchair puts pressure on the same places, making these areas more likely to develop sores. These areas are made worse when the person rubs against bed sheets, or is pulled up in the bed or chair. These open sores, which can expose nerve endings, can become infected causing additional pain if they do not receive appropriate care.

Help Is on the Way

Although we have focused on explaining the causes and types of pain, the good news is that pain is not an inevitable result of cancer. When it does occur, effective treatments are almost always available. Doctors and other medical professionals can help you reduce or eliminate pain using relatively simple and proven measures. For the few situations when pain cannot be completely eliminated, it can usually be reduced to manageable levels. The next chapter will help you explain your pain to your health care providers so that you can get the most effective relief possible. The chapters that follow describe ways to manage pain, side effects, and pain-related situations.

CHAPTER 3

Describing and Measuring Your Pain

Howard first noticed the pain in his ribs on his left side when reaching for a plate in the cupboard. He didn't know what to make of it. He had been receiving hormone treatment for prostate cancer for over four years and because the pain was so vague, he didn't know if this new pain could be related. He wasn't scheduled to see his doctor for another month, and he was unsure he could describe what the pain felt like if his doctor asked.

In most cases, you are the best source of information about your pain, since only you can completely convey information about how bad the pain is, where it is located, which pain control methods work, and which do not. No one else can guess about your pain experience. Studies have found that doctors and nurses rarely rate the level of pain severity the same as patients do, and they more often rate patients' pain as less intense than the patients do themselves. These findings highlight the importance of communication. Your health care team will have no way of knowing or understanding your pain unless you tell them. Because there is no reliable method to objectively measure pain, your health care team and caregivers at home will depend on you to keep them informed about your situation.

The "Language" of Pain

When talking with members of your health care team or other caregivers, it can be very helpful to use words and descriptions that clearly and specifically describe your pain. By communicating with your health care team in a "common language," you can provide reliable and consistent descriptions. This helps them make an accurate diagnosis of the causes of pain and decide which treatment options to prescribe.

In order for you (and others) to get a better understanding of your pain, ask yourself the following questions:

When did my pain begin?

This is also known as the *onset* of your pain. Knowing when the pain first began is important information your doctor can use to determine the source of pain and whether or not it is related to cancer. Pain that began before the diagnosis of cancer may be caused by other, non-cancer sources and may require a different type of treatment. The onset of pain may, on the other hand, be the reason you sought medical advice in the first place and which led to a diagnosis of cancer. You should remember that not all of the pain you experience is necessarily caused by your disease.

How long does my pain last?

Duration describes how long your pain lasts. *Acute* pain appears suddenly (and often with great intensity) and disappears or diminishes quickly as well. Acute pain may be accompanied by rapid heartbeat and an increase in blood pressure. Patients who experience acute pain may wince, grimace, or rub the affected area. Often, acute pain is caused by the cancer itself, such as the swelling of the tumor. In contrast, *chronic* pain is usually less intense but can last for a long time—in some cases many months (see Chapter 2).

Where (in what part of my body) do I feel pain?

Location is where you feel the pain. Sometimes pain starts and remains at a single spot. At other times it can radiate from one point to other parts of the body. The location of pain can change, and sometimes pain in one part of the body indicates that a problem exists elsewhere. For example, gallbladder disease is known to produce pain in the right shoulder. This is known as "referral" pain. The knowledge that pain may arise at sites other than where the problem originates helps clinicians decide on the type of treatment needed.

What does the pain feel like?

Pain *quality* is described by words such as stabbing, burning, crushing, and many other terms. The quality of your pain is yet another factor that provides clues about the source of pain and what measures will be most effective in treating it. The following table contains a wide selection of terms that can apply to pain. Looking at this list may help you to better describe your pain.

Words For Describing Pain

Flickering	Periodic	Pricking	Tingling
Quivering	Intermittent	Boring	Itchy
Pulsing	Jumping	Drilling	Smarting
Beating	Flashing	Stabbing	Stinging
Pounding	Shooting	Lacinating	Dull
Throbbing	Tugging	Hot	Sore
Pinching	Pulling	Burning	Hurting
Pressing	Wrenching	Scalding	Aching
Gnawing	Tender	Searing	Heavy
Cramping	Taut	Tiring	Sickening
Crushing	Rasping	Exhausting	Suffocating
Fearful	Splitting	Wretched	Annoying
Frightful	Punishing	Blinding	Troublesome
Terrifying	Grueling	Cool	Miserable
Spreading	Cruel	Cold	Intense
Radiating	Vicious	Freezing	Unbearable
Penetrating	Killing	Continuous	Nagging
Piercing	Tight	Steady	Nauseating
Brief	Numb	Constant	Agonizing
Momentary	Drawing	Sharp	Dreadful
Transient	Squeezing	Cutting	Torturing
Rhythmic	Tearing	Lacerating	

Source: Adapted from the *McGill Pain Questionnaire*. © 1996 Ronald Melzack. Used by permission.

Is my pain constant, or does it change?

Your doctor or nurse will want to know about the *pattern* of pain, such as how often it comes and goes and whether its intensity, location, or duration changes during the day. They may also want to know whether routine actions, such as moving your arms, breathing, swallowing, standing, sitting or lying down triggers or eases your pain.

How severe is my pain?

Severity, or intensity, is often the most easily described component of pain. Your doctor or nurse may ask you not only to describe the severity of your pain in words (such as mild, moderate, or severe) but also to rate it on a special pain rating scale. For many people, using scales to describe the severity of pain is easier than speaking directly about pain.

Talking About Your Pain with Family Members, Caregivers, and Your Health Care Team

As days went by, Howard's pain became more of a bother to him. His wife of thirty-five years, noticing him grimace while bending over, asked if everything was okay. He told her about the pain in his ribs and how frightened he was that it could be the cancer returning. She decided to accompany him to his doctor's visit.

Just talking about pain can be difficult. For many individuals, knowing how to describe the pain does not make it easier to talk about it, especially with people such as medical personnel. There are many reasons why pain can be a difficult subject. Some patients don't want to seem to be a bother or, worse, don't want to disappoint the doctor. Some feel they are tough enough to live with the pain, while others don't want to admit they have pain for fear that it might mean their cancer has gotten worse or has spread. While some people can talk openly about their pain with a doctor or nurse, others find it easier to begin talking about it by confiding in someone they feel closer to.

Other than yourself, family members and others who care for you are the next best source of information about your pain and the effectiveness of pain treatment. Because caregivers spend more time with you than your health care team, they are in a unique position to observe whether pain treatments appear to be effective and whether they cause side effects. They are most likely to notice any changes in your daily habits or ability to maintain routines, such as eating, sleeping, and moving.

Family members, friends, and caregivers can greatly benefit from an understanding of your experience of pain, what measures relieve your pain, and what factors seem to make it worse. By understanding your experiences, they know what changes to watch for and when to contact your doctor. They can also become important partners by reminding you to take your pain medications on time and by helping you evaluate and describe your pain.

At the doctor's office, Howard's wife went with him into the exam room. "How have you been feeling?" asked the doctor. "Okay, I guess," was his response. "That's not exactly true," said his wife, who proceeded to explain his new pain to the doctor. Based on this information, his doctor ordered several tests. A small growth was discovered on one of his ribs. After discussion with his doctor, Howard and his wife decided he would undergo radiation treatment to the rib to relieve the pain.

For your health care team to most effectively treat your cancer pain, they must understand your experience of it. The information you share provides your health care team with important clues about the source of pain and the best way to provide relief. In addition to the key factors described above, you should let them know what pain treatments have typically worked the best for you in the past, as well as how pain affects your mood and your level of psychological distress.

When you meet with doctors and nurses, let them know your goals and what you would like to happen as a result of your visit. Sometimes complete freedom from pain is a reasonable goal, while at other times getting enough relief to allow you to walk outside or to sleep comfortably at night may be more realistic. Explaining what you need helps them make the best choices regarding your care. Make sure that you convey as much information as possible about your pain, even if some of it seems trivial. Let your health care team decide which details are important and which are not, and remember that no question is stupid or silly when the subject is your health and well being.

If you don't understand something, ask the doctor or nurse to repeat it or explain it more clearly. Good communication between patients and health care providers is known to improve the quality of care that patients receive, and pain relief efforts are more likely to succeed when you describe your pain to the health care team on a regular basis.

Pain should be assessed at every office visit to your doctor or nurse, because the information provides important clues about the progression or regression of disease and the need to change pain control plans. If your pain is causing problems for you, raise the issue when you meet with your doctor or nurse. Make sure that your health care team "hears" you. Don't be afraid to take control of your treatment. During attempts to bring pain under control, you may become frustrated, anxious, or impatient. Express these sentiments to your health care team without fear that they may become angry or upset with you.

Many people find it helpful to take notes or to have a companion take notes for them so they can fully concentrate on the information being discussed and so they won't forget any important information once they return home. After pain treatment begins, regularly updating your health care team about your pain helps them to assess the effectiveness of treatment and the presence of side effects. Such information may prompt your doctor to increase or decrease the dose of your pain medication or to add another medication to your regimen.

Questions to Ask Your Health Care Team About Pain

- What kind of pain am I likely to experience during or after this treatment?
- How do I know whether my pain is "normal" or a sign of some other complication?
- What kind of pain should I watch out for and report?
- Will I need pain medication?
- What kind of pain medication will I need? What are the potential side effects?
- What if the pain medication isn't working? Should I take more?
- Can I become dependent on pain medication?
- How long will I have to take pain medication?
- What options do I have for pain control without medication?
- What else can I do to reduce pain?

When seeking advice over the telephone, list in advance the subjects you want to discuss before calling your doctor or nurse. You may simply have a question about medication dose or timing, or you may be calling to report the onset of new pain. In either case, you can help yourself by being prepared, knowing specifically what information you seek, and by being ready to supply the doctor with important information about your pain, the medications you take as well as how often, and how much relief you currently get from treatment. By supplying this information, you are more likely to avoid delays in treatment.

How Pain Is Measured

Pain assessment is an ongoing diagnostic process during which a member of your health care team (usually a doctor or nurse) evaluates your pain and the effectiveness of pain control measures. According to the guidelines of the Joint Commission on the Accreditation of Healthcare Organizations, hospitals are now required to monitor and document pain levels for all patients (see Appendix B). Patients are asked to rate their pain at all stages of treatment using a numerical scale, so it can be tracked and attended to regularly.

The pain assessment process includes three components: an initial pain assessment; persistent, frequent reassessments as long as pain persists; and routine assessments for the occurrence of new pain. The overall goals of pain assessment are to create a detailed picture of how pain influences different aspects of your life, to identify the cause or causes of your pain, and ultimately to develop an effective pain relief program to match your specific needs.

THE INITIAL PAIN ASSESSMENT

In addition to the radiation treatments, Howard was referred to a nurse specializing in pain management for evaluation. He and his wife prepared a list of questions prior to the appointment. They discussed how he had reacted to pain in the past, and how pain medications might help him in the future if necessary. He was asked to describe his pain in his own words, and to indicate the present level of his pain on a numeric scale so that the specialist could get an idea of the distress he was in. After hearing him describe his pain as a "3" on a scale from 0 to 10, the specialist decided to first try treatment with nonopioid pain relievers. He was instructed to call the office if the pain did not subside within three days.

The initial pain assessment will most likely include a comprehensive medical history that covers information such as your marital and job status, physical activity levels, recreational activities, support networks, social activities, strengths and weaknesses, and spiritual beliefs. The more information your health care team has about you as a whole person, the better able they will be to recommend treatments that might work best for you. You may also be asked if you have a reliable friend or family member who can take you to and from medical appointments and provide care at home, if necessary.

As discussed above, your doctor or nurse will also ask questions about your pain, such as the onset, intensity, severity, quality, location, and the effects the pain has on your physical and emotional well being. If you have been taking pain medications, the assessment will cover their effectiveness. You will also be asked to report all other types of prescription and non-prescription medications you are taking, including herbal supplements or any other complementary or alternative methods you are using.

The initial pain assessment may also include a thorough physical examination to identify any areas of tenderness and to monitor vital signs (such as heart rate and blood pressure), which may increase during periods of pain. Blood tests and other diagnostic procedures, such as x-rays, computerized tomography (CT) scans, and magnetic resonance imaging (MRI), may be ordered. While these tests don't reveal much information about the pain itself, they may indicate changes in bones and soft tissues that can help your doctor identify sources of pain and whether or not cancer cells have spread to other parts of the body. Such information helps health care providers decide on the best course of action to relieve your pain.

Your doctor or nurse may perform a psychological assessment (also known as a psychosocial assessment) to determine how the pain affects your attitudes, mood, and emotions, and what impact it has on your daily activities. Physical pain often causes emotional changes such as anger, anxiety, fear, moodiness, lack of concentration, and depression. You may be asked about your cognitive style, which describes how you view and interpret the world, and whether you experienced any emotional disturbances before your diagnosis, such as depression, anxiety, or moodiness, or whether you are generally overly concerned about health matters. You'll be asked how you typically cope with stress and pain, your expectations about pain management, the meaning of the pain to you and your family, significant past instances of pain and their effects on you, and your concerns about using controlled substances to manage pain. You will also be asked to report any previous or current drug or alcohol usage, which can affect the way a person reacts to pain relief medications.

Your doctor or nurse will also review your cancer history and the current status of your illness and treatment so that they can determine if all or part of your pain is the result of cancer or if it stems from other causes. Not all of the pain you feel is necessarily caused by cancer; it could come from other sources such as injury, bruising, and conditions related to aging, such as arthritis.

From the detailed information that you provide during the initial pain assessment, your health care team can develop a pain relief program tailored specifically to your physical and spiritual needs.

PREPARING FOR A PAIN ASSESSMENT

You can take a number of steps to ensure that you get the most from your pain assessment. One strategy is to review the variety of words for describing pain (see page 47) and select those that best describe your condition. It will also be helpful to write down a complete list of *all* of the medications you take, including the doses, times when you take them, and your opinion about how effective each one is. This list should include any dietary supplements, herbal remedies, and non-prescription medicines that you take. Many doctors recommend packing all of your pill bottles in a bag and taking them with you to the pain assessment.

Consider bringing a friend or close relative to the pain assessment. Ideally, your companion should be the person who is responsible for your overall care at home and who can serve as an advocate for you and provide aid when you are faced with important decisions. Your companion can also help you prepare questions before you go and take notes during the visit so that you can focus completely on the information provided by your doctor or nurse. A friend can also help you review the results of the assessment and make sure that you adhere closely to the plan prepared by your health care team. If you prefer to attend a pain assessment alone, you can benefit from taking careful notes or bringing a tape recorder.

Some doctors or nurses may encourage you to bring family members to the initial pain assessment so they can understand the treatment plan, the importance of controlling pain, and how pain affects your life. They can also learn how to discuss pain with you, be more aware of pain relief needs at home, understand

(continued on page 56)

Suggested Preparation for a Pain Assessment

Before the Assessment

- Write down any questions that come to mind.
- Write down specific goals you expect to reach at the pain assessment. (What do you want to happen as a result of your visit?)
- Ask a companion to accompany you to the pain assessment to lend support and to help you record and interpret important information.
- Bring a pad of paper and a pencil to write down important information.
- Consider tape recording the pain assessment. (Ask for permission ahead of time.)
- List any specific pain-related problems you're having such as limited physical movement or emotional distress.
- Rate the intensity of your pain before and after you take pain medicine.
- Record the times when your pain was worst for several days before your visit.
- List any side effects caused by your medicine or by the pain itself.
- Record any measures, other than medication, you've tried to relieve pain and how well they worked (e.g., complementary pain treatments like hypnosis, relaxation, chiropractic, massage, or acupuncture).
- Make a list of all medications you currently take; include the dosage and the time(s) you take them. (As an alternative, you may want to bring all of your pill bottles with you.)
- For all pain medicines you are taking, list:
  1) the name of the medicine (either the trade name, which is capitalized, or the generic name)
  2) the amount of medicine in each pill (usually listed on the bottle in milligrams, or mg)
  3) how many pills you take for each dose
  4) the time between doses
  5) how much medication you've taken in the past two days
  6) how long it takes the medicine to work
  7) the level of relief the medicine provides
  8) how long the relief lasts
  9) if the pain returns before the next dose, and if so how mild or severe it is

During the Assessment

- Ask for an explanation of any word or phrase you don't understand. Your doctor or nurse should be able to explain medical terms in common language.
- If you don't understand something, ask the doctor or nurse to repeat it. Don't leave the doctor's office until you are satisfied that all of your questions are answered and that you understand the reasons for all treatment decisions.
- Don't be afraid to ask questions, no matter how trivial you think they are. Your questions are valid and important.
- Communicate to your health care team how much and what type of information you want them to give you.
- Tell the doctor or nurse the most effective way for you to receive information, such as through verbal explanations, from written materials, or through pictures. For some people, a combination of methods may work best when learning about complex medical subjects.
- Describe how pain interferes with your daily activities.
- Describe how you feel about the pain (e.g., angry, resigned, sad).
- Have your companion take careful notes, or take notes yourself if you are alone.
- Insist on privacy.

Questions to Expect at a Pain Assessment

- When did your pain begin?
- What does it feel like? Sharp, dull, throbbing? (See page 47 for words to describe pain.)
- Where do you feel your pain?
- Does the location of your pain remain constant or does it move around?
- Is your pain constant? If not, how many times a day (or week) does it occur?
- How long does each period of pain last?
- How severe is your pain?
- Does your pain prevent you from doing your daily activities? Which ones?
- What makes your pain better or worse?
- What have you tried for pain relief and what were the results?
- What have you done in the past to relieve other kinds of pain?
- What medications for pain are you now taking?
- Does your current medication work, and how long does it last?
- Do you notice any side effects from your pain medication?

the effects of various pain medications, how to help you cope with side effects or problems, and when it is necessary to contact a doctor.

The following are tools you can use to get the most from a pain assessment and leave the meeting with all of the information you need to understand the various components of your pain relief program.

Tools for Rating Your Pain

Pain has many dimensions, all of which provide clues about its source and how it can be treated most effectively. There are a number of diagnostic tools available to help you rate and describe your pain.

NUMERIC SCALES

One of the most common types of pain rating tools is called a numeric scale. Numeric scales rely on numbers to help patients describe the intensity of their pain. Scales may range from 0 to 5, 0 to 10, or even 0 to 100, where 0 represents no pain and the highest number represents excruciating pain. Numeric scales can be used verbally or in a visual format (on a sheet of paper). Numbers are often displayed graphically along a line that is divided into segments. Patients can describe their pain level by marking a point along the line or by naming a number that best describes the severity of their pain, for example, "My pain is a 4 on a scale of 0 to 10." Numeric scales are often used to measure pain levels before and after a patient takes pain medication. They are easily understood by patients and generally provide an accurate measure of pain.

Source: Jacox, A. et al. 1994. *Management of Cancer Pain: Adults, Quick Reference Guide for*

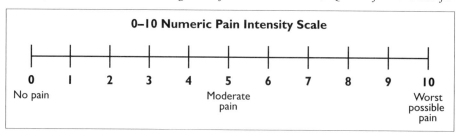

0–10 Numeric Pain Intensity Scale

0 — 1 — 2 — 3 — 4 — 5 — 6 — 7 — 8 — 9 — 10

0 No pain   5 Moderate pain   10 Worst possible pain

Clinicians, Number 9. AHCPR Publications No.94-0593. Rockville, MD: Agency for Health Care Policy Research, U.S. Department of Health and Human Services, Public Health Services.

THE VISUAL ANALOG SCALE

A variation of the numeric scale is the visual analog scale, in which a line is displayed on a page without numbers. The far left end of the line represents "no pain," while the right end represents "pain as bad as it could possibly be." The patient is asked to make a mark along the line that correlates to the amount of pain they are in. While the visual analog scale may be more accurate than numeric scales when used properly, many patients have a difficult time with it and find numeric scales easier to understand. So, this scale is not commonly used.

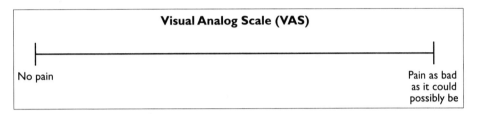

Visual Analog Scale (VAS)

No pain | Pain as bad as it could possibly be

Source: Jacox, A. et al. 1994. *Management of Cancer Pain: Adults, Quick Reference Guide for Clinicians, Number 9.* AHCPR Publications No.94-0593. Rockville, MD: Agency for Health Care Policy Research, U.S. Department of Health and Human Services, Public Health Services.

WORD SCALES

Word scales present a patient with a predetermined continuum of words to choose from, such as "mild," "moderate," or "severe," or phrases such as "no pain," "a little pain," or "too much pain." For some patients, word scales are more effective than numeric scales for rating levels of distress. Word scales have been found to be particularly useful with elderly patients.

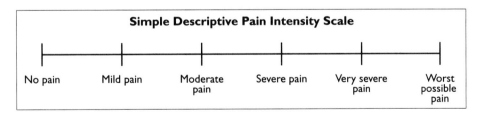

Simple Descriptive Pain Intensity Scale

No pain | Mild pain | Moderate pain | Severe pain | Very severe pain | Worst possible pain

Source: Jacox, A. et al. 1994. *Management of Cancer Pain: Adults, Quick Reference Guide for Clinicians, Number 9.* AHCPR Publications No.94-0593. Rockville, MD: Agency for Health Care Policy Research, U.S. Department of Health and Human Services, Public Health Services.

Another way to rate pain nonverbally is with the faces scale, which consists of a series of faces that are smiling or frowning to various degrees or which show a neutral expression. To use the faces scale, patients point to the expression that most closely reflects their experience of pain. The faces scale is often used for children who are in pain but who cannot verbalize their sensations. It is also a useful tool for adults.

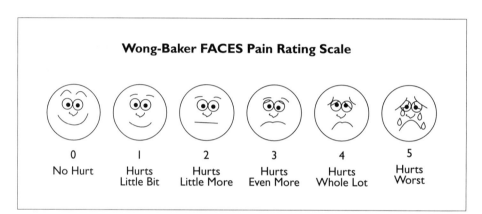

Source: Wong, D.L., Hockenberry-Eaton, M., Wilson, D., Winkelstein, M.L., Ahmann, E., and DiVito-Thomas, P.A., *Whaley and Wong's Nursing Care of Infants and Children, ed. 6,* St. Louis, 1999, Mosby, p. 1153. Copyrighted by Mosby-Year Book, Inc. Reprinted by permission.

Another way to communicate pain level is to select a color from a chart that best reflects the intensity of pain. Scales often begin with white (representing no pain) and end with red (representing severe or excruciating pain). Intermediate colors represent the range of pain levels in between.

All of these types of scales can be useful in helping to answer questions such as:

- How bad is your pain at its worst?
- How bad is your pain most of the time?
- How bad is your pain at its least?

The Brief Pain Inventory consists of questions designed to assess a patient's physical condition and psychological state, which can have a powerful effect on pain. This written form, which takes about fifteen minutes to complete, provides information about pain history, intensity, location, and quality.

Throughout our lives, most of us have had pain from time to time (such as minor headaches, sprains, and toothaches). Have you had pain other than these everyday kinds of pain today?

                    1. Yes   2. No

On the diagram, shade in the areas where you feel pain. Put an X on the area that hurts the most.

Right   Left   Left   Right

Please rate your pain by circling the one number that best describes your pain at its *worst* in the last 24 hours.

0   1   2   3   4   5   6   7   8   9   10

No
Pain   Pain as bad as
you can imagine

Please rate your pain by circling the one number that best describes your pain at its *least* in the last 24 hours.

0   1   2   3   4   5   6   7   8   9   10

No
Pain   Pain as bad as
you can imagine

Please rate your pain by circling the one number that best describes your pain on the *average*.

0   1   2   3   4   5   6   7   8   9   10

No
Pain   Pain as bad as
you can imagine

6. Please rate your pain by circling the one number that tells how much pain you have *right now*.

0   1   2   3   4   5   6   7   8   9   10

No
Pain

Pain as bad as
you can imagine

7. What treatments or medications are you receiving for your pain?

_____

_____

8. In the last 24 hours, how much relief have pain treatments or medications provided? Please circle the one percentage that most shows how much relief you have received.

0%   10%   20%   30%   40%   50%   60%   70%   80%   90%   100%

No
relief

Complete
relief

9. Circle the one number that describes how, during the past 24 hours, pain has interfered with your:

A.   General Activity

0   1   2   3   4   5   6   7   8   9   10

Does not
interfere

Completely
interferes

B.   Mood

0   1   2   3   4   5   6   7   8   9   10

Does not
interfere

Completely
interferes

C.   Walking Ability

0   1   2   3   4   5   6   7   8   9   10

Does not
interfere

Completely
interferes

D.   Normal Work (includes both work outside the home and housework)

0   1   2   3   4   5   6   7   8   9   10

Does not
interfere

Completely
interferes

E.   Relations with Other People

0   1   2   3   4   5   6   7   8   9   10

Does not
interfere

Completely
interferes

F.   Sleep

0   1   2   3   4   5   6   7   8   9   10

Does not
interfere

Completely
interferes

G.   Enjoyment of Life

0   1   2   3   4   5   6   7   8   9   10

Does not
interfere

Completely
interferes

What to Do After the Initial Pain Assessment

Following the radiation treatment and daily doses of Vioxx (a long-acting, aspirin-like medication), Howard's pain was diminished but still bothersome. He had difficulty getting out of bed without discomfort, and was unable to pick up his young grandchildren without experiencing sharp pangs in his ribs. His wife phoned his doctor's office, and he was scheduled for a return visit. His doctor placed him on a stronger analgesic. Within a week his pain was all but gone.

Once a pain assessment has been completed, pain relief measures should begin immediately if possible. Pain should not be an excuse for failing to complete a careful diagnostic workup, since the results will determine the course of action that will relieve discomfort.

There are a variety of medications and other methods including complementary non-medical treatments your doctor may recommend (see Chapter 7). Often, pain relief medications are prescribed in combinations to enhance their effectiveness. The sedative effects of many pain medications are enhanced by alcohol. Combining alcohol with prescription pain medicines (e.g., opioids) and anti-inflammation medications (e.g., ibuprofen) can be dangerous. Even small doses may cause problems. Some nonprescription medications, such as those for allergies, may also increase the sedative effects of opioids. Be sure that your doctor knows about all of the medications you take and whether you can continue to use them after beginning therapy for pain.

After beginning treatment for pain, it is important to stay in close touch with your health care team to report the results, or lack of results, of your treatment. If your pain level does not seem to decline in the expected time or if the relief is inadequate, call your doctor. Don't wait for your next scheduled appointment to report your situation. Your doctor may increase the dose of your pain medication to increase its effectiveness or switch you to another medication or combination of medications.

THE PAIN LOG

You may find it helpful to keep a record or diary to track the onset, duration, location, quality, patterns, and severity of pain you are experiencing. Filling out a daily pain log allows you to bring an accurate history of your pain to your next

	Time of pain onset	Duration	Location	Quality	Triggers	Severity
Monday						
Tuesday						
Wednesday						
Thursday						
Friday						
Saturday						
Sunday						

meeting with your health care team. This can help them to monitor any trends in your pain as well as how well pain treatment is working for you.

Follow-up pain assessments should be conducted on a regular basis and should be scheduled every time you experience a new type of pain or if an existing pain grows worse or changes noticeably in character. During follow-up pain assessments, your health care team will evaluate the effectiveness of pain relief measures that were initiated after previous pain assessments. Based on the information you provide, your doctor will determine if changes in your pain status are related to the progression of disease or to cancer treatment and then decide if any changes (such as trying a new pain medication or increasing the dose of a current medication) should be made to your pain management plan.

As mentioned earlier, communication between patient and doctor or nurse is one key to successful pain management. The more detail you can provide during a pain assessment, the greater the chances that the pain relief program prescribed by your doctor will decrease pain and improve the quality of your life in the short-term and the long-term. Friends or family members can offer opinions about your pain experience based on their observations, but the person in pain remains the best and most reliable source of information about his or her experiences.

Only you know whether a certain pain medication works or doesn't and whether you can tolerate side effects if they occur.

Your health care team should regularly monitor your pain and the effects of medication, but you must play a role to ensure that you receive adequate attention and the highest quality of care. In general, you should communicate any changes in your physical, emotional, and psychological condition after beginning pain medication. If pain medication doesn't work, make sure you inform your caregivers and a member of the health care team. Depending upon your goals, the doctor may discuss with you the possibility of raising the dose of the successful medication to bring additional relief. Communication and perseverance are crucial in making sure you receive the most effective combination of pain medications and doses. Only after numerous options involving pain relief medications have been explored will your doctor consider more intensive measures.

Assessment for Recurrence of Pain

Once your pain is under control, you and your caregivers must be watchful for signs of its return. Pain can reappear in an old location, but it is important to

Notify Your Doctor If:

- You experience any new or severe pain.
- You are unable to take anything by mouth, including pain medication.
- The pain causes you to cry out, become still, or double over.
- You have any questions about how to take your medications or if new symptoms accompany your pain (such as inability to walk, eat, sleep, or urinate).
- You are unable to sleep because of pain.
- You have decreased appetite because of pain.
- You cry, feel upset, feel helpless or feel depressed because of your pain.
- You notice new areas of redness or swelling in an area of pain.
- Your prescribed pain medicines do not relieve the pain or do not relieve it for long enough.

realize that new areas of the body may also become involved over time, and new pain may have a different quality from what you experienced in the past.

If you experience the onset of new pain, increased severity of existing pain, or side effects you suspect may be caused by pain medications or other treatments, do not hesitate to tell caregivers or contact your doctor. The more quickly you inform others about a change in your pain status, the more quickly steps can be taken to control pain and reduce side effects. There is no way of knowing whether the pain will go away on its own and nothing will be gained by "waiting it out." Suffering in silence may seem noble and independent, but it is unnecessary and doesn't accomplish anything. Pain can and should be treated whenever it causes discomfort or interferes with your life.

CHAPTER 4

Pain Relief Through Medication

"Mary was admitted to the hospital unit where I worked. She had back pain and went to surgery for a ruptured disc. She did not have a disc problem but instead had a large malignant tumor wrapped around her spine. Following her surgery, Mary's doctor treated her back pain with Demerol (meperidine). The medical oncologist, who was asked to see Mary, knew Demerol was effective for surgical pain but not for chronic cancer pain. Mary's pain was caused by the cancer pressing on the nerves in her back and not the surgery. I watched the medical oncologist change her pain medicine and quickly increase the dose until Mary had some relief. She pointed to the crying face when asked how bad her pain was. The crying face soon changed to a frown with no tears. This told us that Mary's pain was beginning to be relieved. With continued adjustment of her pain medicine, and adding other medicines to help, it was so rewarding to see Mary's face change to no frown and no tears, then to what appeared to be a smile. As I continued to be involved in Mary's care, I began to realize that relieving Mary's pain was how we could help Mary the most. I learned a lot from Mary. She was a turning point in my life. There was something about Mary that directed my career to oncology nursing."

Terri, a cancer nurse

Cancer pain can be treated in a variety of ways, including treating the underlying cancer with surgery, chemotherapy, and radiation. The use of medicines, known as drug therapy, is the cornerstone of pain treatment. Drug therapy brings significant relief in most cases, regardless of a patient's age or whether pain is acute or chronic. Relieved of pain, people with cancer often resume normal activities and enjoy an improved quality of life.

The goal of pain therapy is straightforward: to avoid pain that can be prevented and to control pain that cannot, while limiting medication-related side effects. Many doctors place a great deal of importance on making sure a patient can sleep pain free. Adequate sleep not only increases tolerance to pain, it also boosts energy levels during the day and improves overall well being. Ensuring that patients can be comfortable while at rest (but awake) or when moving is also an important consideration.

As a rule, your doctor will match the type and amount of pain medication to the severity of your pain. Mild pain relievers, many of which do not require a prescription, are often used for mild cancer-related pain. If pain gets worse, your doctor will most likely prescribe more potent drugs. Often, medications are combined to enhance pain relief or to relieve drug-related side effects. Other important factors to consider are your previous experiences with pain, the success of any previous drug therapy for pain relief, the type of cancer treatment being used, and the doctor's familiarity with the medications.

Pharmacologic therapy (the use of drugs) is the foundation of cancer pain relief. In 90 percent of people with cancer, pain can be controlled with few side

What's in a Name?

When discussing drugs, remember that every medication has two names: the generic name, which describes the chemical content of the drug, and the brand name, which is the name the drug is sold under. Typically, the brand name is capitalized while the generic name is written in all lower case letters. A single generic drug may be marketed under several brand names. For example, the generic drug aspirin is sold under numerous well-known brand names, such as Bayer and Ecotrin. The generic drug acetaminophen is probably best known by the brand name Tylenol, though it is also sold under other brand names. And the generic drug ibuprofen is marketed under several brand names, including Motrin, Advil, and Nuprin. The generic name of a drug is printed somewhere on the label of a brand name medication. Some generic drugs are sold without any brand names attached. For instance, you can purchase a bottle of generic ibuprofen or generic acetaminophen. Generic drugs typically cost less than brand name products.

effects. Decisions about which drugs to prescribe, at what dosages and frequencies, are guided primarily by the severity and character of the patient's pain, the patient's tolerance level of pain, and the risk of and potential for medication-related side effects. The goal is to achieve the greatest amount of pain relief in the simplest manner while minimizing drug-related side effects.

Drugs used to relieve pain are called analgesics, which act on various parts of the nervous system to relieve pain without causing loss of consciousness. Analgesics provide only temporary relief, which is why they must be taken regularly to effectively decrease or eliminate symptoms.

Three-Step Analgesic Ladder for Cancer Pain Management

Not all people with cancer will experience pain, and those who do are not in pain all of the time. Although there are ways of controlling pain through medication, some people suffer needlessly rather than ask their doctors to prescribe stronger medication or change their medication. Some even believe pain is just something they have to "deal" with. Pain can negatively impact work, sleep patterns, appetite, and other daily activities, leading to a lower quality of life for the person with pain. But, it does not have to. To guide doctors and other health professionals who treat cancer pain, the World Health Organization (WHO) developed the *Three-Step Analgesic Ladder for Cancer Pain Management*, which is summarized below. The steps on the ladder and the recommended relief match the severity of pain a person is having.

STEP ONE: MILD PAIN – NONOPIOID DRUGS

The first step of the pain ladder calls for nonopioid drugs to relieve mild pain, such as the drug acetaminophen or one or more drugs from a large group of pain medicines, known as nonsteroidal anti-inflammatory drugs (NSAIDs). Among the most well-known NSAIDs are aspirin and ibuprofen. Your doctor may also prescribe an adjuvant pain medication, which is used either to enhance the effects of the analgesics or provide relief for specific types of pain.

Adjuvant pain medicines are medicines that have some other primary purpose than relieving pain, but when used with pain medicines, they are effective in helping to relieve some of the pain. They may be used during all three steps

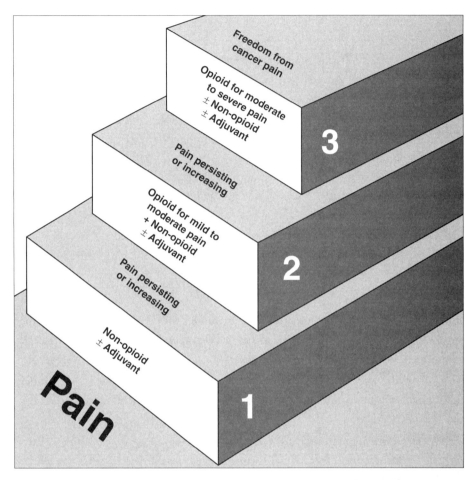

Source: The World Health Organization Three-Step Analgesic Ladder for Cancer Pain Relief. From *Cancer Pain Relief and Palliative Care*. Report of a WHO Expert Committee. Geneva, Switzerland. © 1990 World Health Organization. Used by permission.

of the pain ladder and include antidepressants (such as Elavil), anticonvulsants (such as Tegretol or Dilantin), and corticosteroids (such as dexamethasone and prednisone). Once the medicine is started, you should notice some decrease in pain within a few days of using the adjuvant medicine. If you do not, or if you notice other side effects, you should tell your doctor or nurse. Your doctor may increase your dosage or switch you to a different adjuvant medicine.

STEP TWO: MODERATE PAIN – "MILD" OPIOID DRUGS

If acetaminophen or NSAIDs with or without adjuvant medications do not provide sufficient pain relief or if their effects do not last long enough, your treatment will move to the second step of the pain ladder. At this point, your doctor is likely to continue your NSAID therapy but will add to it a mild opioid (narcotic) drug. Typical examples of mild opioids include codeine (sold under numerous brand names) and dextropropoxyphene (Darvon, Darvocet). More popular for pain relief nowadays are oxycodone (Percodan, Percoset) and hydrocodone (Vicodin, Lortab). Sometimes, mild opioids and NSAIDs are combined in a single pill. Adjuvant medications may also be prescribed along with mild opioids to enhance pain relief.

STEP THREE: SEVERE PAIN – STRONG OPIOIDS

The last step on the pain ladder calls for the use of strong opioids to control severe pain that can not be controlled with mild opioids or mild opioids in combination with NSAIDs and adjuvant medicine. Morphine is considered the "gold standard" against which all other cancer pain treatments are measured because it is such an effective pain reliever.

There are a number of strong opioids doctors can choose that vary somewhat in their side effects. Some opioid pain medicines are also available in "sustained release" (long-acting) forms that last for eight or twelve hours, such as MS Contin or Oramorph (morphine products) or OxyContin (oxycodone). Kadian is a slow-release morphine pill that lasts for up to twenty-four hours, and Duragesic is available as a patch that delivers the drug continuously through the skin for seventy-two hours. As in steps one and two of the pain ladder, the use of NSAIDs or adjuvant medicines are likely to continue to enhance pain control.

If strong opioids alone, or in combination with other drugs, are still not sufficient to relieve pain, other treatments such as surgery and direct anesthetic techniques such as nerve blocks may be needed (see Chapter 5). However, drug therapy is effective in controlling 80 to 90 percent of cancer patients' pain.

HOW TO READ A DRUG LABEL

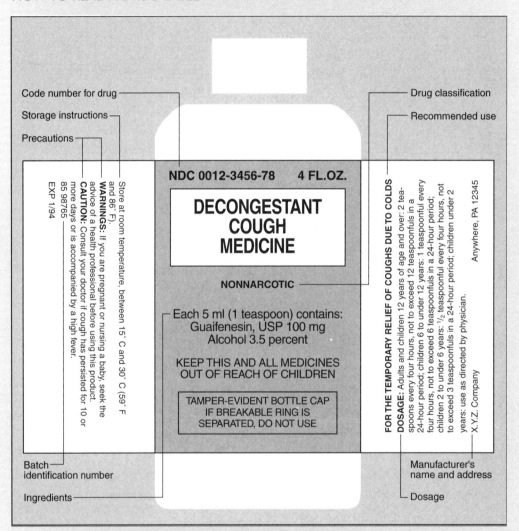

Code number for drug

Storage instructions

Precautions

Drug classification

Recommended use

NDC 0012-3456-78   4 FL.OZ.

DECONGESTANT COUGH MEDICINE

NONNARCOTIC

Each 5 ml (1 teaspoon) contains:
Guaifenesin, USP 100 mg
Alcohol 3.5 percent

KEEP THIS AND ALL MEDICINES
OUT OF REACH OF CHILDREN

TAMPER-EVIDENT BOTTLE CAP
IF BREAKABLE RING IS
SEPARATED, DO NOT USE

Store at room temperature, between 15˚ C and 30˚ C (59˚ F and 86˚ F).
WARNINGS: If you are pregnant or nursing a baby, seek the advice of a health professional before using this product.
CAUTION: Consult your doctor if cough has persisted for 10 or more days or is accompanied by a high fever.
85 98765
EXP 1/94

FOR THE TEMPORARY RELIEF OF COUGHS DUE TO COLDS
DOSAGE: Adults and children 12 years of age and over: 2 teaspoons every four hours, not to exceed 12 teaspoonfuls in a 24-hour period; children 6 to under 12 years: 1 teaspoonful every four hours, not to exceed 6 teaspoonfuls in a 24-hour period; children 2 to under 6 years: ½ teaspoonful every four hours, not to exceed 3 teaspoonfuls in a 24-hour period; children under 2 years: use as directed by physician.
X.Y.Z. Company   Anywhere, PA 12345

Batch
identification number

Ingredients

Manufacturer's
name and address

Dosage

Used with permission from *Nurse's Fact Finder*, 1991, © Lippincott, Williams & Wilkins.

Drugs Used for Controlling Cancer Pain

NONSTEROIDAL ANTI-INFLAMMATORY DRUGS (NSAIDS)

NSAIDs are the mainstay of drug therapy on the first step on the pain ladder, but they are also likely to be used during steps two and three as well. NSAIDs do their work outside of the central nervous system by inhibiting, or stopping, the actions of a chemical called prostaglandin. Some types of prostaglandins are responsible for causing pain. By slowing down the rate of prostaglandin production, NSAIDs dull pain receptors and reduce pain. NSAIDs also reduce inflammation and by doing so, reduce pain caused by inflammatory processes.

There are about twenty different kinds of NSAIDs, including ibuprofen (see Appendix A). Chemically, they are similar, but the effectiveness may vary with different medicines. Some popular NSAIDs are widely advertised and you are likely to recognize brand names such as Advil and Nuprin. Generic versions of the same products are often available at a lower price. Some NSAIDs that are available over-the-counter require a doctor's prescription at higher dose levels.

The first medication you take for pain control may not be the most effective. Keep a positive outlook because there are many drugs in the NSAID family from which your doctor can choose. Finding out which one is most effective for you is often a matter of trial and error. Your doctor may first prescribe an NSAID that you remembered worked well in the past. The only way to know if one NSAID is more effective than another for relieving pain is to try it out and gauge the results. One NSAID may effectively relieve pain for one person, whereas another type may not, so trying different drugs in the NSAID family can be helpful in finding the most effective medication.

If your doctor chooses an NSAID that is available without a prescription, it doesn't mean that the NSAID won't work to relieve your pain. NSAIDs can be surprisingly effective and are much stronger than many people realize. In many cases, NSAIDs are all that is needed to relieve cancer pain. This is especially true if patients "stay on top of the pain" by taking the medicines on schedule and not waiting until the pain returns. It is easier to manage pain by taking the medicine on a regular schedule in the absence of pain than by waiting until the pain becomes troublesome. Researchers evaluating the effects of NSAIDs for cancer pain have found these drugs often provide sufficient pain relief for many, but that their effectiveness is limited in people with advanced cancer.

Types of Pain Relief Medicines

Analgesics can be categorized broadly into two groups:

- Nonopioid medicines used for mild to moderate pain
- Opioid medicines used for moderate to severe pain

Many nonopioid pain relievers may be purchased "over-the-counter" without a doctor's prescription; others require a prescription. An opioid is a narcotic that is chemically related to opium or synthetic forms of opium. (The word "narcotic" comes from the Greek term for numbness.) All opioid pain relievers require a doctor's prescription.

Stomach upset and indigestion are the most common side effects of NSAIDs. Taking them with food or milk, or immediately following a meal lessens such responses. NSAIDs can also cause vomiting, constipation, and bleeding in the stomach. If your stools become darker than normal or if you notice blood in your stool—both signs of bleeding in the gastrointestinal tract— tell your doctor or nurse. In addition, some people with bleeding or clotting disorders may not be able to take NSAIDs because of the effect of the medicines on the blood's ability to clot. People who are receiving chemotherapy drugs that can lower their blood platelets may be cautioned against taking NSAIDs during specific times of their chemotherapy cycle.

Other potential side effects of NSAIDs are dizziness, headache, ringing in the ears, fluid retention, dry mouth, and increased heart rate. NSAIDs may also produce kidney problems and stomach ulcers. Some NSAIDs can cause liver damage and for this reason, people taking these medicines should limit their intake of alcohol.

Each NSAID has a maximum dose that can be taken at one time. Medicines given beyond this limit produce no additional pain relief, but increase the risk of side effects. You should take no more than the prescribed or recommended dose. While receiving NSAIDs, you will be monitored closely for potential side effects. Laboratory studies involving blood tests will be done on a regular basis.

ACETAMINOPHEN

Acetaminophen is a well-known nonopioid pain reliever that is similar to NSAIDs but which does not reduce inflammation. Acetaminophen is typically used during the first step of the pain ladder, but may be continued during the second step. The drug may be given alone or in a pill combined with a mild opioid (Tylenol III is one example). Side effects associated with acetaminophen are rare. Liver or kidney damage, however, may result among those who take large doses daily for a long period of time or who regularly drink alcohol with the usual dose.

Your doctor may ask that you not take acetaminophen regularly or during specific times during your treatment if you are receiving chemotherapy. Since one of the side effects of many chemotherapy drugs is lowered white blood cell counts which can result in infection, the doctor will want to be able to watch for signs and symptoms of infection which include a fever. Taking acetominophen will mask the presence of a fever, which may be a sign of infection that requires immediate treatment.

OPIOIDS

Opioids are similar to natural substances produced by the body (endorphins) to control pain. These medicines were once made from the opium poppy, but today most are synthetic—that is, made by drug companies. See Appendix A for detailed information on specific opioids and other pain relief medicines.

Unfortunately, opioids have wrongly been associated with illegal "street" drugs. Furthermore, myths and misunderstandings have led to the underuse of opioids in many cases where patients in significant pain would greatly benefit from them. But, opioids are exceedingly effective in relieving cancer pain. Increasingly—in large part because of the experience gained from the hospice movement in England—health care professionals are recognizing the benefits of opioid analgesics for treating cancer pain.

Opioids can be given alone, and they are often prescribed in combination with nonopioid analgesics (i.e., NSAIDs or acetaminophen) as well as with other adjuvant medications. Opioids are usually given by mouth, but for patients who have difficulty swallowing or who have significant side effects from taking opioids by mouth, these drugs can also be given intravenously or into a vein, as rectal suppositories, or through a number of other drug delivery systems (see pages 81–86). Opioids are available in both short-acting and time-release forms with effects that may last for many hours.

NSAIDs Aren't for Everyone

In general, NSAIDs should be avoided by people who:
- Are allergic to aspirin
- Are on chemotherapy (anticancer drugs)
- Are on steroid medicines
- Have stomach ulcers or a history of ulcers, gout, or bleeding disorders
- Are taking prescription medicines for arthritis
- Are taking oral medicine for diabetes or gout
- Have kidney problems
- Will have surgery within a week
- Are taking blood-thinning medicine

Individuals may experience mild side effects when taking opioid medications (see Chapter 6). The most common side effects are predictable and usually manageable by either altering the dose or prescribing medications to control the side effects. Typical side effects include sedation (drowsiness), constipation, nausea, and vomiting. Some people may also experience dizziness, mental effects (nightmares, confusion, hallucinations), decreased rate and depth of breathing, difficulty in urinating, or itching.

Mild Opioids

If nonopioid analgesics do not bring sufficient pain relief within twenty-four to forty-eight hours, your doctor is likely to add a mild opioid to your treatment regimen. Codeine is one example of a mild opioid. Many people who take opioids benefit from continuing to take regular doses of NSAIDs or acetaminophen.

Because the two types of drugs attack pain in distinct ways, combining them often enhances pain relief. NSAIDs cut off the pain signal at the site of pain, while opioids block the signals passing through the central nervous system and decrease the sensitivity of pain receptors.

For many patients, mild opioids in combination with NSAIDs are sufficient to prevent or control pain. The dose of mild opioids is increased until adequate pain relief is achieved. As with NSAIDs, finding the most effective opioid pain reliever is often a matter of trial and error.

When to Get Immediate Help for the Side Effects of Pain Medicines

A drug reaction is a different type of emergency related to pain control. People may be allergic to pain medicines, or the pain medicines may be too strong. Call the doctor or nurse immediately if any of the following symptoms occur when taking pain medicines:

- Hallucinations
- Ringing or buzzing in the ears
- Confusion or being "out of it"
- Great trouble waking up even when others try to wake the person
- Severe trembling, uncontrolled muscle movements or convulsions (seizures)
- Unable to hold in urine or stool when this was not a problem in the past
- Nausea or vomiting with no relief
- Hives, itching, skin rash, or swelling of the face
- Feeling anxious or "fidgety"
- Slow breathing (fewer than eight breaths per minute) or very shallow breathing (short breaths that don't take in much air)

Strong Opioids

When pain becomes severe and does not respond to mild opioids, stronger opioids are usually needed. Strong opioids are the most powerful and most effective pain relievers. The best known strong opioid is morphine. Morphine is frequently the first choice for treating pain, especially for the elderly or patients with severe cancer-related pain. A number of brand name drugs contain morphine or morphine-like chemicals (Morphone, MS Contin, Oramorph). Other frequently used strong opioids include hydromorphone (Dilaudid), levorphanol (Levo-Dromoran), methadone (Dolophine), and oxycodone (Oxycontin, Percodan, Percocet). Your doctor is likely to continue to prescribe NSAIDs and adjuvant medication along with a strong opioid.

Treatment with strong opioids is begun at low doses under careful medical observation. The dose is raised until pain relief is achieved or until side effects become a problem. If one drug is not effective or if the patient is particularly sensitive to its side effects, the doctor may try another drug. The new drug will probably be prescribed at a dose equivalent to that of the last opioid, since the patient has already had time to adjust to the effects of opioids in general.

Although it was once believed that strong opioids were not very effective when given by mouth, today the oral route is preferred. Morphine and other strong opioids given orally appear to work extremely well at all dose levels, though other routes of administration are necessary for some patients.

Doctors carefully adjust the doses of opioids so there is little possibility of overdose. Therefore, it is important that two different doctors do not prescribe opioids for you unless they first talk with each other. Tell any doctors you deal with if you drink alcohol or take tranquilizers, sleeping aids, antidepressants, antihistamines, or any other medicines that make you sleepy. Combining opioids with these substances can be dangerous, even at low doses, and can lead to an overdose with symptoms of weakness, difficulty in breathing, confusion, anxiety, and severe drowsiness or dizziness.

Other Types of Pain Medications

ADJUVANT ANALGESICS

Adjuvant means used in addition to the primary treatment. With cancer pain, medicines are prescribed to enhance the effects of NSAIDs or opioids. These are called adjuvant analgesics. Adjuvant medicines are used to treat some other illness but in the presence of cancer pain, they are used along with a primary cancer pain medicine. Though some research shows a few adjuvant drugs possess pain relieving qualities, they are rarely used alone for pain control.

The following table is an overview of the major classes of adjuvant medicines that might be prescribed to enhance pain relief. (See Appendix A for more detailed information on specific medications.)

Antianxiety Drugs

Cancer patients commonly become anxious during exams and treatment. Severe anxiety can interfere with a person's ability to function, decrease the ability to comprehend, and increase painful sensations. Anxiety may be linked directly to pain, in which case a painkiller may reduce both. Antianxiety drugs,

Drug Class	Generic Name	Trade Name	Action	Side Effects
Antianxiety drugs	diazepam, alprazolam, lorazepam, haloperidol	Valium, Xanax, Ativan, Haldol	Used to treat anxiety and also to treat muscle spasms that often go along with severe pain.	Drowsiness. May cause urinary incontinence.
Anticonvulsants	carbamazepine, clonazepam, gabapentin, phenytoin	Tegretol, Klonopin, Neurontin, Dilantin	Helps to control tingling or burning from nerve injury caused by the cancer or cancer therapy.	Liver problems and lowered number of red and white blood cells. Gabapentin may cause sedation and dizziness.
Antidepressants	amitriptyline, nortriptyline, desipramine, doxepin, fluoxetine, paroxetine, sertraline	Elavil, Tofranil, Pertrofrane, Sinequan, Prozac, Paxil, Zoloft	Used to treat tingling or burning pain from damaged nerves. Nerve injury can result from surgery, radiation therapy, or chemotherapy.	Dry mouth, sleepiness, constipation, drop in blood pressure with dizziness or fainting when standing. Blurred vision. Urinary retention. Patients with heart disease may have an irregular heartbeat.
Corticosteroids	dexamethasone, prednisone,	Decadron, Prednisone	Helps relieve bone pain, pain caused by spinal cord and brain tumors, and pain caused by inflammation. Increases appetite. Relieves nausea associated with chemotherapy.	Fluid buildup in the body. Increased blood sugar. Stomach irritation. Sleeplessness. Mood changes.

such as mild tranquilizers, can help people feel calmer and counter the anxiety-producing effects of some pain medications. Tranquilizers are also prescribed for people who experience panic attacks. Patients who don't respond to tranquilizers may require stronger antianxiety medications, such as haloperidol (Haldol), which may reduce confusion and agitation.

Side effects of tranquilizers include drowsiness, confusion, and uncoordinated movements. Patients using tranquilizers should avoid alcohol, because the combination can lead to extremely dangerous side effects.

Anticonvulsants

Anticonvulsants (antiseizure medicines), such as carbamazepine (Tegretol), phenytoin (Dilantin), clonazepam (Klonopin), and gabapentin (Neurontin), are used primarily to control convulsions (e.g., seizures associated with epilepsy). But as adjuvant medicines, they may also relieve sharp stabbing, shooting, burning, or tingling pain caused by tumors pressing on nerves, especially in the head and neck. Such pain can be difficult to treat with opioids alone. Anticonvulsants are occasionally prescribed to reduce pain following surgery and for people with limb amputation, stump pain, or pain in the lower extremities.

Antidepressants

Some standard (tricyclic) antidepressants may be used to relieve tingling and burning pain. For example, Amitryptyline (Elavil, Endep), doxepin (Adapin, Sinequan), and imipramine (Tofranil) all demonstrate the ability to reduce neuropathic pain, which is a dull, burning sensation caused when cancer cells invade or press on nerves. Tricyclic antidepressants have also been used to control pain caused by mastectomy and other surgeries. The most notable side effects associated with tricyclic antidepressants include dry mouth, constipation, low blood pressure, and sedation, all of which can be troublesome for patients using opioids. More recently developed antidepressants (i.e., selective serotonin reuptake inhibitors, such as Prozac, Paxil, and Zoloft) may also be used to reduce depression experienced by many people who live with pain, but they are not used to treat pain directly.

Corticosteroids

Corticosteroids (also called steroids) reduce swelling, inflammation, and pain caused by tumors that press on or invade nerves or bones. Steroids also can promote appetite and improve mood. The drug dexamethasone (Decadron) is commonly used to treat back pain due to spinal cord compression. Prednisone (Deltasone) is a common choice for treating patients who have advanced cancer. People with advanced cancer who receive steroids often need lower doses of opioids to control pain. Corticosteroids may also be used as a treatment for certain cancers.

Steroids can cause a number of undesirable and potentially dangerous side effects, such as adrenal insufficiency, which is characterized by loss of appetite, nausea, dizziness, depression, low blood sugar, and low blood pressure. Adrenal insufficiency can be fatal. It can also cause fluid retention which can lead to high blood pressure and heart failure, low calcium, low potassium, osteoporosis, and increased susceptibility to infections and delay in healing. Because of these risks, corticosteroids are often used for short-term use to control flair-ups of acute pain.

Anesthetic Treatments

Anesthetic techniques, such as nerve blocks, are used to treat cancer pain that is not relieved by other techniques (see Chapter 5). For example, neuropathic pain caused by invasion or compression of a nerve may not be easily relieved by pain medicines given by mouth. Most anesthesia techniques block nerves. For example, pain in the chest wall and abdominal wall can be relieved by interrupting the nerves that exit from the spinal cord to supply these sites. Pain in the legs, groin, and lower back can be helped by giving drugs into the epidural or intrathecal spaces of the spine to numb the nerves that receive pain signals from these sites (see page 84). Patients with upper abdominal pain from pancreatic cancer can get good relief from interruption of the nerves near the pancreas.

Both opioid medicines and local anesthetics are used for this method of pain relief. Morphine and fentanyl are the medicines used most commonly for intrathecal administration. A combination of opioids and anesthetic agents, such as bupivacaine and ropivacaine, are used especially in patients who have not received adequate relief with opioids alone.

A continuous epidural infusion is used when the pain is difficult to treat, as in cases of advanced metastatic disease involving the pelvis and lower body. An infusion pump delivers the pain medicine to the spinal column through a catheter, or a small reservoir is surgically implanted in the body to dispense the drug in small doses over time. The advantage of this method is that it provides effective relief without disrupting the function of the muscles and nerves.

Side effects resulting from medicines given into the spine include urinary retention, itching, nausea, vomiting, and decreased respirations.

Clinical Trials

Clinical trials, or studies involving patients, are the mechanism through which advances are made in cancer treatment. Through these studies, more effective and safer treatments have been found that have contributed largely to the decrease in cancer death rates in the United States. These clinical studies look at ways to improve cancer treatment, but also study ways to improve patients' quality of life by improving treatment of side effects such as nausea and vomiting, mouth sores, and pain control. The development of continuous pain medication infusion pumps (patient-controlled analgesia, see pages 85–86), first developed in the early 1980s, is one example of how advances in treatment have improved the treatment of pain control.

Clinical trials provide the necessary information for the U.S. Food and Drug Administration (FDA) to use in determining whether a new drug shows "substantial evidence of effectiveness," or whether an already approved drug can be used effectively in new ways (for example, to treat other types of cancer, or to give at a different dosage). The FDA must certify that a drug has shown promise in laboratory and animal studies before human testing can begin. The clinical trials process includes three main stages and involves continuous review, which ensures that the sponsor can stop the study early if major problems develop or unexpected levels of treatment benefit are found. As with all clinical trials, benefits and risks must be carefully weighed by the researchers conducting the study and the patients who decide to participate.

Many cancer clinical trials are funded by the National Cancer Institute (NCI) through cancer centers or cooperative networks made up of research institutions, university and community hospitals, and clinics. In addition to the cancer treatment being studied, these institutions also conduct quality of life studies, looking for better ways to improve patients' quality of life by providing appropriate supportive care such as adequate pain control. Pharmaceutical companies often work with university medical centers to study cancer and pain medicines as well. Although these companies have an interest in proving that a medication works, they must follow strict scientific rules for research. For more information about current clinical trials on pain control medicines, contact NCI's Cancer Information Service at 1-800-4-CANCER (1-800-422-6237) or visit their web site at: http://cancertrials.nci.nih.gov.

Methods Used for Drug Delivery

Most pain medicines are taken by mouth, usually as tablets, capsules, or gelcaps. They are usually taken with a large glass of water or other liquid unless your doctor tells you otherwise. Do not take your medicine with alcoholic beverages. Oral medications may cause problems for patients who have difficulty swallowing, or they may cause side effects such as nausea and vomiting. In such cases, your doctor may try a different way to administer the medicine, such as through a skin patch or a suppository, or by injection under the skin or into a muscle or vein.

During the course of an illness, most people need to take pain medications by multiple methods. This is important because the way drugs are administered can make a big difference in their effectiveness. For example, medications given orally or rectally may take longer to work, but they may last longer than medications given intravenously.

ORAL

As a rule, chronic pain is best treated orally. Compared with other drug delivery methods, the oral route is the easiest, least expensive, safest, and generally provides the longest relief. Oral medications also free people from reliance on tubes, poles, and other equipment that hinders mobility, so they can participate more fully in life. Drugs taken orally are generally given in higher doses than those given by other means, because the drug must pass through the stomach's acidic environment before being absorbed into the bloodstream. This method is convenient and relatively inexpensive. However, patients must remember to take these medications on schedule, and as the dose is increased, they may have more pills to swallow.

Oral medications are used when the patient can swallow and the digestive system functions normally. For patients who cannot eat solid foods or have trouble swallowing pills, some pain medicines are available in liquid form, which may be ingested more easily. A pharmacist can also mix a liquid syrup containing one or more pain medicines. Some opioids, including morphine, are available in high concentration elixirs, which can be given in very small volumes.

TRANSMUCOSAL

When a patient cannot swallow tablets or liquid, some medications are taken by putting them inside the cheek or between the cheek and gums. The medicine is absorbed through the lining of the mouth. This route of administration is called transmucosal, meaning that the medicine is absorbed through the mucous lining of the mouth. This is also a favored method for those patients who have difficulty swallowing. However, bitter flavors, irritation, and poor absorption often limit their usefulness.

SUBLINGUAL

Other medications are taken by putting the drug under the tongue for absorption. This route of administration is called sublingual. This method can be used for patients who are unable to take oral medicines. Many hospices use liquid morphine this way for patients who cannot swallow.

TRANSDERMAL (SKIN PATCH)

The transdermal method uses a bandage-like skin patch that releases medicine through the skin and into the bloodstream. The medicine enters the body slowly and steadily for up to seventy-two hours and allows for flexible dosing. Transdermal administration is particularly useful for patients who are already taking strong opioids but are unable to swallow them, who may experience nausea and vomiting after chemotherapy, or who have a blockage in their intestines. Skin patches are usually placed on the chest or back.

Getting to the right dose using this method of administration takes some time. The maximum dose is limited. Another fast-acting medicine (orally or rectally) is often required to treat breakthrough pain. The patch is not suited for those needing quick dose changes. The patch may need to be changed every forty-eight hours.

RECTAL SUPPOSITORIES

Rectal suppositories are often used when a person cannot swallow pills, experiences nausea and vomiting after taking pain medications orally, or is unable to eat or drink before surgery. Once placed in the rectum, a suppository melts and releases the drug into the body. The process is painless and generally causes only minimal discomfort for most people. Opioids and nonopioids are available as suppositories. Suppositories can also be placed through abdominal openings (called stomas) made during surgery for colorectal cancer.

This is a simple, safe, and low cost method. However, suppositories must be avoided if there are sores in or around the rectum. They cannot be used if a patient has diarrhea or hemorrhoids. Some elderly or disabled people might need assistance using them and some people simply don't like this route of administration.

INJECTIONS

Intravenous (IV) Injections and Intravenous Lines

With intravenous injections, drugs are delivered through a needle or thin plastic catheter directly into large veins in the arm. With an IV, a needle or thin catheter is placed into a large vein in the arm and remains there. (When IV lines are inserted into large arm veins, they are called Hickmans, Broviacs, or peripherally inserted central catheters.) Both IV injections and infusions are suitable for patients who have constant nausea and vomiting, cannot swallow, have mouth and throat pain, and are confused or have mental status changes that prohibit swallowing medicines. They are also useful for delivering very high doses of medication or when dose changes are needed quickly and are made often. They provide a constant and rapid onset of pain relief. With IV lines, patients do not require an injection every time drugs are given. The IV tubing protrudes from the skin a few inches and dressings are changed as needed.

Implanted ports are a new way to deliver medicine into a large vein in the chest. These circular, metal ports are about one inch wide and one inch deep. Ports are usually surgically placed under the skin of the upper chest. A nurse locates its exact placement by gently pushing on the skin and feeling the small round disc where the medicine is to be injected into the port. The nurse cleans the skin with a solution and injects medicine into the port, which flows into the vein. This method provides easy IV access without frequent injections into a vein. There is some risk of infection, so this route is used only when less invasive methods are not available.

Intramuscular (IM) Injection

Using a syringe, medications may be injected directly into muscle tissue. This route is useful for pain control if the patient can't take oral medicines and the IV route is not available. This allows for the medication to work quickly. However, it is difficult to predict how long the medicines will be effective, and IM injections are painful so they are generally discouraged.

Subcutaneous (SQ or SC) Injection and Infusion

With subcutaneous injections, drugs are delivered with a syringe just beneath the skin. With subcutaneous infusion, a small needle is implanted just under the skin. Every few hours, the patient or a caregiver can give medicines manually through tubing connected to the implanted needle. Alternatively, an automated pump can be hooked directly to the implanted needle to inject medication on a preset schedule. With this delivery method, patients do not have to receive an injection every time medication is needed.

Intraspinal Injections

With this method, drugs are injected either into the epidural space, which is the space between the bones of the spine and the outer layer of the spinal cord, or into the intrathecal space of the spinal canal, which is the space just outside the spinal cord. Opioids are more potent when given into the intrathecal space as compared to the epidural space. Intraspinal injections are used when the patient's cancer pain is responsive to opioids but when the side effects are too great to be tolerated when given IV or by mouth. When given directly into the central nervous system, the medicines do not affect the entire body, so there are fewer side effects.

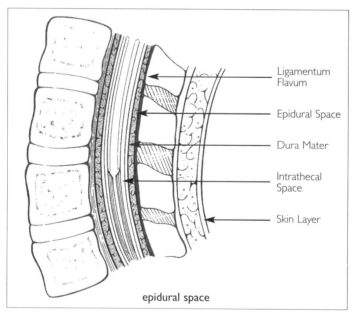

Source: Management of Cancer Pain with Epidural Morphine. An Independent Study Module. ©2001 SIMS Deltec. Used by permission.

PATIENT-CONTROLLED ANALGESIA

One of the newer approaches to cancer pain management allows patients to control the administration of medicines at a rate and dosage that they choose. This method is referred to as patient-controlled analgesia, or PCA, and is very common in many cancer care facilities.

PCA (sometimes called demand or self-administered analgesia) uses an electronic infusion pump attached to a drug reservoir and a timing device. A tube is connected to a small needle or thin plastic catheter inserted under the skin (SQ) or into a vein (IV). When patients feel pain, they press a button on the pump and receive a preset dose of medication. The timer is adjustable so that no more than a certain amount of drug can be taken over a given time. PCA is often used after surgery or for anyone with severe pain.

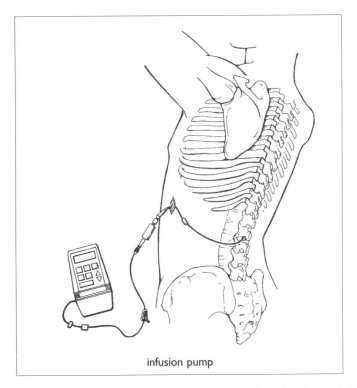

infusion pump

Source: Management of Cancer Pain with Epidural Morphine. An Independent Study Module, ©2001 SIMS Deltec. Used by permission.

Some studies suggest that patients who control their own medication tend to be discharged earlier after surgery and may suffer fewer chronic pain problems later. Patients who control pain themselves may use lower total doses of the drug than would have been prescribed by doctors. Most people prefer this arrangement to receiving injections every few hours. If nothing else, PCA offers a psychological advantage, because pain is often easier to bear if you know you can relieve it whenever you want.

Today, miniature pumps are available that fit into a fanny pack, backpack, or purse and deliver a continuous infusion of analgesic medication.

Managing Your Drug Therapy Program

The first step in developing a drug therapy plan is to talk with your health care team about your pain. Every patient's drug therapy plan will be different, because the way each person deals with pain and reacts to various medications varies considerably. What works for one person may be completely unsuitable for another. You can help ensure that you end up with the appropriate drug therapy plan by communicating openly, honestly, and frequently about your pain and the effects of medication. Be sure to inform your health care team about all types of prescription and non-prescription medications you are taking, including herbs, vitamins, and other supplements.

The most effective way to control pain with drugs is to keep symptoms at bay and prevent them from returning. For this reason, it is important for you to closely follow your medication schedules, even if you are not in pain, and pay attention to when it's time to take the next dose. Once pain re-emerges, it becomes much more difficult to control. Following your doctor's directions about when and how much medication you take is important to the success of your drug therapy program. Get in the habit of regularly informing your doctor or another member of your health care team how well your medications are working so that your therapy can be altered if necessary.

If the first attempt at pain control using drugs does not succeed, don't be discouraged. As mentioned earlier, your doctor has many options from which to choose, including increasing the dose of a prescribed medication, switching to a stronger medication, or prescribing multiple medications. Often, doctors must

How to Get the Most from Your Medication Plan

There is no single choice of medicines in general for any one person, nor is there any such thing as a standard dose of opioids. Each person has a different threshold for tolerating pain and the effects of medications, and each will have different treatment needs. Your doctor or pain specialist will determine the appropriate starting dose. Here are several guidelines you can follow to get the most benefit from your drug therapy program:

- Take your pain medication on schedule as prescribed by your doctor to help prevent persistent or chronic pain.
- Do not skip doses of your scheduled medicine. Once you feel pain, it is harder to control.
- If you experience "breakthrough" pain, use your short-acting medicine as your doctor suggests. Don't wait for the pain to get worse.
- Never stop or start taking pain medications without first checking with your doctor or nurse.
- Be sure only one doctor prescribes your pain medicine. If a second doctor changes your medicine, the two doctors should discuss your treatment with each other before you take the new prescription.
- Never take someone else's medication. Medicines that worked for you in the past or helped a friend or relative may not be right for you and may pose risks when combined with other drugs.
- Remember that pain medicines affect different people in different ways. A very small dose may work for you, while someone else may need to take a much larger dose to obtain the same level of pain relief.
- Keep a record of your pain and pain relief (see pages 96–97).
- Remember that your pain control plan can be changed at any time.

experiment with drug therapy before they find the best combination. Many factors must be considered when prescribing drugs, including your age, tolerance of pain and side effects, and desired level of activity. Sometimes a medication may provide adequate pain relief but also cause unpleasant side effects. Ideally, drug therapy will relieve pain without causing undue side effects, but sometimes these two opposing results must be weighed against each other.

If you need to be taken off opioid medications, your doctor will advise gradually cutting back to minimize the uncomfortable symptoms of withdrawal, which may include flu-like symptoms, agitation, sleeplessness, fear, worsening of pain, and excessive perspiration. Tell your doctor immediately if you experience any of these symptoms. They can be treated and tend to disappear within a few days or a few weeks, but it is best to avoid withdrawal altogether by decreasing the dose of opioids slowly.

CONTROLLING BREAKTHROUGH PAIN

It is common for people with persistent pain to experience episodes of breakthrough pain as well. Breakthrough pain is a brief and often severe flare of pain that occurs even though a person may be taking pain medicine regularly for persistent pain (see Chapter 2). If you have breakthrough pain, it does not mean that the pain medicine you are using regularly is not working well. It occurs even when a person is taking the correct dose of pain medicine on a regular schedule for persistent pain.

Breakthrough pain is best treated with medicines that work quickly and for short periods of time. This is different from persistent pain medicines that work for long periods of time. Breakthrough medicines are usually given on an "as needed" or "prn" basis, which means that they are taken when you have breakthrough pain. These short-acting medicines (sometimes called "rescue" medicines) work faster than the medicines you are using for your persistent pain, so that you can get pain relief sooner. They also stay in your body for a shorter period of time in order to cause fewer side effects.

The most common medicine used to treat breakthrough pain is immediate-release morphine given as tablets, capsules, or liquid. Other medicines for breakthrough pain that promise faster and more effective pain relief are currently being developed. Ask your doctor or nurse about your treatment options for breakthrough pain.

Why Doctors May Prescribe
Two Different Opioid Pain Medicines

Since persistent pain and breakthrough pain are different types of pain, they can be treated with different pain medicines. Persistent pain is usually treated with long-acting medicines that are taken regularly to prevent as much pain as possible. Breakthrough pain is relieved with short-acting medicines that are taken only when you have episodes of breakthrough pain.

The pain medicines that you have been prescribed work together to treat both your persistent pain and breakthrough pain. Your persistent pain medicine takes longer to work, but it helps to control your pain for hours to days. When you experience breakthrough pain, your breakthrough pain medicine works faster but for a shorter period of time to directly control the flares of breakthrough pain.

It is important that you take the short-acting medicine when you first begin to feel breakthrough pain, so it can begin to work to relieve the pain. Do not let the pain build up and become too severe because then it will be much harder to control. You may also want to take a dose of your breakthrough medicine if you know that you are likely to have breakthrough pain with a particular activity. Follow the directions given to you. If the labeled dose does not relieve your breakthrough pain or if you think you are having too many episodes of breakthrough pain, contact your doctor or nurse. They may need to adjust the dose or frequency of your breakthrough pain medicine.

There may be times when you experience breakthrough pain right before or after taking your persistent pain medicine. At these times, you should take your breakthrough pain medicine and continue to take your persistent pain medicine according to your regular schedule. You should always follow the directions given to you by your doctor or nurse. It may be helpful to mark your medicine bottles clearly "for breakthrough pain" or "for regular pain." If you find that you are regularly having breakthrough pain right before your usual dose of persistent pain medicine, you should talk to your doctor or nurse. They may need to adjust the dose or the frequency of your persistent pain medicine.

Taking two different opioid pain medicines will not cause more side effects. In fact, a long-acting and short-acting medicine are both given so that you will have fewer side effects. Most people only have breakthrough pain a few times a day, and the breakthrough pain is usually much more severe than their persistent pain. By taking a short-acting medicine for breakthrough pain, you are getting the extra medicine when you need it. Generally, you can expect the same types of side effects from your breakthrough pain medicines as from your long-acting medicines.

If your breakthrough pain medicine is not relieving your breakthrough pain, if you are having breakthrough pain more than four times a day, or if you have any questions about when to take your persistent pain or breakthrough pain medicines, contact your doctor or nurse.

WHEN TO NOTIFY YOUR DOCTOR

If you have chronic cancer pain and are taking medicines to control your pain, call the doctor or nurse immediately if any of the following conditions exist:

- You experience any new or severe pain.
- You are unable to take anything by mouth, including pain medication.
- Your prescribed pain medicines do not relieve the pain or do not relieve it for long enough.
- You become constipated, nauseated, or confused.
- You have any questions about how to take your medications or if new symptoms accompany your pain (such as inability to walk, eat, sleep, or urinate).
- You are unable to sleep because of pain.
- You become so groggy that it's difficult to carry on a conversation or stay awake.
- You cry, feel upset, feel helpless, or feel depressed because of your pain.
- You experience hallucinations (seeing things that aren't actually there).
- You feel disoriented.
- You are unwilling to move, or muscles are very tense when moving.
- The pain is constant, remains in one spot or gets stronger.
- The pain causes you to cry out, become still, or double over.
- You notice new redness, swelling, or pus.
- You get hives, itches, or a rash.
- You experience uncontrolled muscle movements (twitches or jerks).

- You have decreased appetite because of pain.
- Pain continues to be a problem in between doses of long-acting medicines.
- Pain interferes with your normal activities, such as eating, sleeping, working, and sexual activity.

Tolerance, Dependence, and Addiction

Many people worry that they will get "hooked" on opioids and won't be able to stop taking them. This is one of the greatest misconceptions about opioids and one that often results in the underuse of pain medications. Patients who take opioids to relieve pain are not addicts nor are they at serious risk of becoming addicts no matter how much of the drug they take or how often they take it. Opioids are powerful drugs that should be used only under a doctor's supervision, but the fear of addiction is unfounded. Yet many people with cancer still fear opioids, and some health care professionals resist prescribing them, even when they are most needed.

DRUG TOLERANCE

People who take opioids for medical reasons often find that larger and larger doses are needed to achieve the same level of pain relief. This may be the result of increased pain or a phenomenon known as drug tolerance. Drug tolerance occurs when your body adjusts to a medication and it does not relieve pain as effectively as it used to. Not all patients experience drug tolerance, but it is a common occurrence.

If tolerance occurs, the correct medical strategy is to increase the dose or to change to a different opioid medication. *Neither strategy leads to dependence or addiction.* Unlike the nonopioid analgesics, opioids have no maximum dose and sometimes large amounts of a drug are needed to achieve adequate pain relief.

Many doctors and nurses still do not understand that tolerance differs from addiction. The two are completely different and should not be confused. Yet misinformation about opioids leads some health care professionals to limit or stop their use when they notice a patient is becoming drug tolerant. Some believe that if "too much" of a drug is used now, the medication will not work later when the patient "really needs it." This assumption is incorrect. People in pain may benefit from opioids at any given point during their pain experience.

The Myths About Opioids

- **"Opioids pose a strong risk of addiction."** False. The risk is less than one in 3,000. Unfortunately, the misplaced fear of addiction often means that these drugs are not used as frequently as they should be, or in the right doses, to provide adequate pain relief.
- **"Opioids produce euphoria, which inevitably leads to being hooked."** Not true. People taking opioids for pain relief seldom report feeling euphoric. Even if they do, it is unlikely that they will continue to seek drugs for their euphoric effects after the pain has abated.
- **"People are given morphine only when they're at death's door."** No. In good cancer management opioids are administered as soon as pain becomes moderately severe. As the ladder strategy suggests, opioids are appropriate treatment when nonopioids alone fail to provide the amount and duraton of relief the person needs.
- **"Morphine doesn't work when taken by mouth."** False. This belief originated from some faulty studies done some years ago. In fact, oral morphine is very effective. (However, injected opioids may work faster at lower doses.)
- **"Heroin is a better opioid than morphine."** Untrue. The body converts heroin to morphine.
- **"People always need high doses of opioids."** Wrong. Every person is different. Effective doses of morphine can range from 5 to 180 mg every four hours. Most people require only moderate doses; in fact many people with advanced cancer and chronic severe pain need no more than 20 mg every four hours, no matter how long the therapy lasts.

DRUG DEPENDENCE

There are two kinds of drug dependence: physical dependence and psychological dependence. Neither is the same as drug tolerance. *Physical dependence* is normal and predictable, and it is not a very serious result of using opioids. Anyone who takes a high enough dose of an opioid for a long enough time is likely to become physically dependent on it. The most obvious signs of dependency are

- **"I'll die of an overdose."** Not likely. Many people fear opioids because of news reports about drug users who die of overdoses. Even though the doses required for adequate pain relief are sometimes high, they are rarely if ever, large enough to cause death. Among substance abusers, death usually results when they take outrageously high doses or consume dangerous combinations of substances, like a heroin-and-cocaine "cocktail." And addicts often take illegal opioids manufactured by amateur scientists, compounds that contain impurities or are "cut" with adulterating substances such as talcum powder.

- **"There's a limit to the effective dose of an opioid."** Not so. The stronger the pain is, the more is required for relief. Again, NSAIDs do have a ceiling dose, but opioids can be used in increasing amounts until they bring the pain under control. Furthermore, increasing the dose (often a necessary step in managing the pain of progressive cancer) does not increase the already minimal risk of addiction.

- **"People taking opioids always need to take antivomiting drugs."** Some do, especially in the beginning. Women are more prone to experience vomiting. But in most cases, the antivomiting therapy can be stopped after a few days.

- **"People should take morphine only when they feel the need."** No, The best strategy is to take regular doses around the clock, rather than on an as needed, or p.r.n., basis.

withdrawal symptoms that appear when a person suddenly stops taking a drug. Withdrawal symptoms include agitation, fear, chills, sweating, shaking, sleeplessness, and worsening pain. Though withdrawal is an unpleasant experience, it can easily be avoided and well managed if opioid doses are reduced gradually over time. Physical dependence *is not* addiction.

Psychological Dependence and Addiction

When trained health professionals refer to addiction, they are speaking of *psychological dependence*. Addicts take drugs to satisfy physical, emotional, and psychological needs, not to treat medical problems. An addict's life is centered on obtaining and taking drugs, despite the financial, legal, or health consequences. Using an opioid is only one factor in developing a psychological dependence. Other important variables include a person's social, economic, and psychiatric background. Though it is possible for patients who takes opioids for pain to become psychologically addicted, the risk is incredibly small, especially among patients with no history of substance abuse. The *Journal of the American Medical Association (JAMA)* reported that pain is often not adequately treated because of the fear that increased use of opioids can lead to abuse.[1] However, the study found that the increased medical use of opioids has not lead to an increase in abuse of the drugs.

Changing Your Pain Medicine or Drug Therapy Plan

If one medicine or treatment does not work, there is almost always another one that can be tried. Also, if a schedule or way that you are taking medicine does not work for you, changes can be made. Talk to your doctor or nurse about finding the pain medicine or method that works best for you. You may need a different pain medicine, a combination of pain medicines or a change in the dose of your pain medicines if:

- Your pain is not relieved.
- Your pain medicine does not start working within the time your doctor said it would.
- Your pain medicine does not work for the length of time your doctor said it would.
- You have breakthrough pain.

[1] D. E. Joranson, K. M. Ryan, A. M. Gilson, and J. L. Dahl, "Trends in Medical Use and Abuse of Opioid Analgesics," *JAMA*, 283 (2000): 1710–1714.

- You experience serious side effects such as trouble breathing, dizziness, and rashes. Call your doctor right away if these occur (Side effects such as sleepiness, nausea, and itching usually go away after your body adjusts to the medication. Let your doctor know if these bother you).
- The schedule or the way you are taking the medicine does not work for you.

In addition to changing medications, your doctor can choose other strategies to improve your pain treatment:

Increase the dose of medicine. Sometimes there is not enough medicine in the body to prevent pain. If so, your doctor may increase the dose until adequate pain relief is achieved.

Shorten time between doses. The right amount of pain medication may not remain in the bloodstream because the drug isn't taken often enough. If so, your doctor may shorten the time between doses. You can help to determine if this is a problem by writing down the time you take pain medication and how long afterwards the pain returns.

Use short-acting or immediate-release opioids for breakthrough pain. If you experience breakthrough pain while taking your regular, long-acting pain medicines as prescribed, your doctor can prescribe special doses of pain relievers that work very quickly. Sometimes people need to have their dose of pain relievers almost doubled to prevent breakthrough pain from happening again.

Use a medication in a different form or with a different delivery technique. In addition to being given by mouth, medicines can be administered in a number of other ways, such as intravenously (into a vein), through a skin patch, and through a rectal suppository (see pages 82–83).

Use radiation therapy. Sometimes radiation therapy is prescribed to shrink a tumor that is causing pain (see Chapter 5).

Refer you to a pain clinic. Universities and large hospitals have special clinics to evaluate and treat chronic pain. Pain clinic staffs are specially trained to manage pain using a variety of techniques, including nerve blocks that stop the pain for a short time until other methods are prescribed. Most pain clinics require a doctor's referral.

Pain Records, Charts, and Logs

To treat pain optimally, it is important to gather as much information as possible during pain treatment. Without writing down their experiences, most people have trouble remembering in detail when they experience pain, the nature of the pain at any particular time, what they did for it, or what they were doing when it occurred. Keeping a pain log allows patients to document pain and actions taken to relieve it, including drug therapy. Ideally, a daily pain log not only tracks pain levels, but also helps patients, caregivers, and medical staff understand the effects pain has on you, what steps work best to ease pain, and the best times of day to take pain medications. A pain log can also indicate whether certain physical activities are closely associated with pain and need to be curtailed. Sometimes a pain log indicates clear patterns of improvement after only a few days of regular recording.

WHAT TO INCLUDE IN A PAIN RECORD

Items that may be included in a pain log include:

- A pain rating scale that describes your pain before and after using a pain relief medicine.
- The name and dose of the pain medicine you take.
- How long the pain medicine works.
- The time you take pain medicine.
- Any activity that seems to be affected by the pain or that increases or decreases the pain.
- Any activity that you cannot engage in because of the pain.
- Any pain relief methods used, other than medicine, such as rest, relaxation techniques, distraction, meditation, or imagery.

By tracking the particular time of day you felt pain, what medication you took for it, what nondrug techniques you tried, and your emotional state, you will be able to more clearly convey your particular pain control needs to your doctor, nurse, or caregiver. The following is a sample pain log that may be used to track your pain throughout the day.

Time	Severity from 0 (no pain) to 10 (severe)	Description of how pain feels	What you were doing when it began (e.g., walking, sleeping)	Name and amount of medication taken	Nondrug techniques you tried (e.g., meditation, heat)
Midnight					
1 a.m.					
2 a.m.					
3 a.m.					
4 a.m.					
5 a.m.					
6 a.m.					
7 a.m.					
8 a.m.					
9 a.m.					
10 a.m.					
11 a.m.					
Noon					
1 p.m.					
2 p.m.					
3 p.m.					
4 p.m.					
5 p.m.					
6 p.m.					
7 p.m.					
8 p.m.					
9 p.m.					
10 p.m.					
11 p.m.					

PAIN LOG

CHAPTER 5

Other Methods of Pain Relief

Bruce was sixty-eight years old when he began having abdominal pains and noticed the whites of his eyes taking on a yellowish hue. After several tests at the doctor's office and the local hospital, he was diagnosed with pancreatic cancer. A CT scan showed that the head of the pancreas was pushing against his small intestine, and several large tumors were present in his liver and in other parts of his abdomen. He was started on oral morphine to control his pain but was still uncomfortable even when other pain medications were added.

Oral pain medication is the simplest, least invasive, most versatile, and often most effective method of relieving cancer-related pain. In most cases, patients experience significant pain relief from one or more oral analgesic medications. Of course, treating the cancer itself is an important way to relieve pain and other symptoms of cancer.

For at least 10 percent of patients, however, oral analgesic therapy does not provide sufficient relief. Even after many attempts to find the most effective analgesic combinations and dosages, medications may not adequately relieve pain or may cause intolerable side effects. When analgesic therapy fails to relieve pain adequately, doctors may turn to more invasive and complex methods of pain control.

Palliative Therapy for Pain Control

The three most commonly used primary cancer therapies are radiation therapy, surgery, and chemotherapy. Primary therapies are those directed against the cause of the pain—that is, the cancer itself. Each method may be used alone or in combination with another in an attempt to cure the cancer. However, these therapies can also be used to relieve pain, increase comfort, and improve the patient's quality of life when curative therapy is no longer given. This is known as palliative therapy. Doctors can almost always treat cancer symptoms, such as pain, by using some form of palliative therapy. In addition to the three types of therapy listed above, hormonal therapy and treatment with bisphosphonates may also be used to palliate, or help control, cancer pain.

Patients who undergo palliative therapy usually continue to take pain medications until the effects of the new treatment become evident. Some patients may continue to take them if palliative therapy is not completely effective in relieving their pain.

PALLIATIVE RADIATION THERAPY

Tumors often cause pain when they get large enough to press on surrounding nerves. Radiation therapy can be used to shrink such tumors, which can reduce pain. Often a single dose of radiation therapy is all that is needed to relieve pain. Doctors also use palliative radiation to relieve symptoms such as bleeding, difficulty swallowing, intestinal obstruction (blockage of the intestines), compression of blood vessels or nerves by tumors, and potential fractures that could occur as a result of cancer that has metastasized (spread) to bones.

Radiation treatment sometimes enhances the effectiveness of analgesic medicines and other noninvasive therapies because it directly targets the cancer causing the pain. Treatment is supervised by a radiation oncologist, a doctor who specializes in the use of radiation for cancer patients.

The success of palliative radiation depends on factors such as the type and location of the cancer, as well as the radiation energy source, dose of radiation, and length of treatment. Several methods of radiation therapy are available.

External Beam Radiation

External beam radiation requires a radiotherapy machine that emits high-energy rays capable of killing cancer cells. The radiation oncologist calculates the dose of radiation needed to kill cancer cells while causing the fewest side effects, and then focuses the beam of radiation on cancer cells, even when they are deep inside the body. External beam radiation may involve multiple treatments over several days or weeks.

Internal Radiation (Brachytherapy)

Another method of delivering radiation involves placing small pellets or metal rods containing radioactive materials into or next to a tumor. Each pellet is about the size of a grain of rice and is placed so that the small amount of radiation each one produces can do the most damage to cancer cells while sparing healthy surrounding tissue. The pellets are usually implanted during a simple surgical procedure. This method is called internal radiation, interstitial radiation, or brachytherapy. Sometimes both internal and external beam radiation therapies are used together for palliative purposes.

Radiopharmaceuticals

A radiopharmaceutical is a medicine that contains a radioactive substance. It is injected into a vein to travel to areas where cancer has spread. The radiation emitted by the drug kills cancer cells, thereby relieving pain. This type of radiotherapy is used primarily to treat patients whose pain results from bone metastases. For patients whose cancer has spread to many bones, injection of radioactive medicines is far more effective than aiming external beam radiation at each affected bone. Sometimes a single injection can bring extensive pain relief within a week, and the effects often last for several months. This procedure can be repeated if bone pain returns. In some cases, radiopharmaceuticals are used together with external beam radiation aimed at the most painful bone metastases. This approach has helped many men with prostate cancer, but its usefulness against other cancers is not as well documented. Examples of radiopharmaceuticals include strontium-89, iodine-131, rhenium-186, and samarium-153.

Will I Become Radioactive?

Even though the effects of radiation are powerful, you will not become permanently radioactive. External radiation therapy affects targeted cells only for a moment. With internal radiation therapy, your body may or may not emit a small amount of radiation for a short time. Precautions are taken anyway and may include hospitalization and limitation of visitors. Pregnant women, whose fetuses are vulnerable to the smallest doses of radiation, are not allowed to visit.

Patients who are given radioactive substances such as iodine, phosphorus, or strontium by mouth or into a vein are kept isolated until their bodies no longer contain enough radioactivity to be hazardous to others. Be sure to discuss any safety concerns you have and precautions you need to take with your radiation oncologist, nurse, or the radiation safety officer at your treatment facility.

Side Effects of Radiation Therapy

Dose levels of radiation used for palliative treatment are lower than those used for primary treatment of cancers, so side effects are generally mild. Still, patients may experience a variety of undesirable reactions to radiation therapy (see Chapter 6).

External beam radiation may cause skin to mildly burn or tan. Both effects gradually fade. If the neck area is treated with external beam radiation, the thyroid gland may be damaged, requiring the patient to take thyroid hormone replacement pills. Radiation directed to the head and neck may damage the salivary glands, resulting in dry mouth, sore throat, hoarseness, difficulty swallowing, partial or complete loss of taste, and temporary fatigue. Radiation of the abdomen can lead to nausea, diarrhea, vomiting, and temporary or permanent damage to the intestines. Chest radiation may cause lung scarring that can lead to shortness of breath. Radiation therapy directed at the brain may cause subtle problems with thinking, but the extent depends on the dose used and may not occur until years after treatment.

While radiopharmaceuticals initially travel throughout the body after injection, potential side effects are basically limited to a few areas. Some patients experience a "flare" or increase in bone pain, several days after the injection, which subsides after a few days. Because these drugs tend to concentrate in the bones, the bone marrow may be affected, which can lead to anemia and to an increased risk of bleeding or infection. These drugs are removed from the body through the urine, so some patients may develop cystitis (inflammation of the bladder).

While Bruce's condition was not curable, his doctor explained to him that chemotherapy might shrink the cancer and relieve some of his symptoms. After two cycles of chemotherapy with gemcitabine, he needed less medication each day to control his pain, and the whites of his eyes returned to normal. A CT scan showed that the cancerous tumors were now about half their original size. He underwent two more cycles of chemotherapy, after which the tumors appeared to remain the same size. Because the cancer was no longer shrinking, his doctor decided to give him a break from the chemotherapy, as he had been experiencing severe diarrhea.

PALLIATIVE CHEMOTHERAPY

While surgery and radiation therapy are generally used to treat localized cancers, chemotherapy is used to treat cancer that has spread or metastasized to other parts of the body. Depending on the type of cancer and its stage (extent of spread in the body), chemotherapy can be used to cure cancer, to keep the cancer from spreading, to slow the cancer's growth, or to kill cancer cells that may have spread to other parts of the body. Chemotherapy drugs may also be used as palliative treatment to relieve pain caused by growing tumors or to relieve other symptoms caused by cancer. Palliative chemotherapy is not effective for all patients, and pain relief with this method is usually slow, if it occurs at all.

The anticancer drugs used in chemotherapy are most often given by injection into a vein, or by mouth (in pill form). They enter the bloodstream and travel to all areas of the body. Often, a combination of anticancer drugs is used.

Chemotherapy is usually given in cycles. Each cycle consists of one to several days of treatment followed by a period of three to four weeks to allow the body to recover. Then another cycle of treatment is started, and so on. The total course of chemotherapy is usually four to six cycles, which can last from three to five months, although some chemotherapy regimens are longer.

Chemotherapy can be used as an adjuvant (addition) to surgery in some cases. After a cancer is removed by surgery, chemotherapy can significantly reduce the risk of cancer returning. The chances of cancer returning and the

Palliative Uses of Radiation Therapy

- Relieve bone pain, especially that caused by metastasis from breast, lung, or prostate cancer.
- Relieve pain caused by tumors pressing on or invading nerves.
- Control bleeding caused by tumors.
- Reduce pain caused by tumors that ulcerate, such as certain breast cancers, head and neck cancers, and skin cancers.
- Ease breathing problems (dyspnea), coughing, or chest pains caused by tumors that block the breathing passages.
- Reduce pain caused by large abdominal tumors.
- Relieve pain from tumors that press on the spinal cord or that cause back pain, leg weakness, shooting pains, sphincter problems, or numbness.
- Relieve headaches caused by inoperable brain tumors that press on the skull.
- Shrink tumors blocking hollow organs or tubes, such as the bronchial tubes, esophagus, bile ducts, ureters, lymph channels, blood vessels, gynecologic system, or gastrointestinal tracts.
- Relieve problems caused when the tumors grow in small, constricted spaces.

potential benefit of chemotherapy depend on the type of cancer and other individual factors.

Side Effects of Chemotherapy

Side effects of chemotherapy depend on the type of drugs used, the amount taken, and the length of treatment. Some of the most common side effects are nausea and vomiting, fatigue, temporary hair loss, mouth sores, and increased chance of bleeding and infections. The side effects of chemotherapy can also lead to other types of pain (see Chapter 6). Some side effects may be harder to cope with, while others may be mild. Most side effects can be controlled with medications, supportive care measures, or by changing the treatment schedule.

HORMONAL THERAPY

Hormones are chemical messengers that regulate many functions in different parts of the body. Some types of cancer, especially breast, prostate, and endometrial cancer, grow in response to hormones normally circulating in the blood. In these types of cancer, drugs can be given to lower certain hormone levels, which can slow or stop tumor growth. Sometimes different hormones must be combined before cancer responds, and results might take several weeks to become apparent. Hormonal therapy is palliative in nature—that is, it cannot cure cancer. However, the treatment is capable of providing enduring pain relief without causing some of the more serious side effects seen with chemotherapy. Because hormonal therapy lowers the levels of the major male or female hormones, side effects are often related to sexual function (such as impotence in men and vaginal dryness in women). Hot flashes are also common.

BISPHOSPHONATE THERAPY

Bisphosphonates are a group of drugs that slow down the action of bone cells called osteoclasts. Osteoclasts are cells that normally eat away small pieces of bone, allowing other cells to reform the proper shape of the bone. When cancer spreads to the bones, osteoclasts may become overactive, which can lead to bone pain. Bisphosphonates are used to treat pain in the bones from multiple myeloma as well as from breast or prostate cancer. They are usually given in cycles similar to those used for chemotherapy, although their side effects are less severe.

Three months after the completion of his chemotherapy, Bruce began to notice the yellow returning to his eyes and in the skin of his face as well. The abdominal pain was again difficult to control with pain medication. A CT scan showed that the head of the pancreas had grown again and was preventing the liver from emptying its bile into the intestines, which was causing his jaundice. After consulting with his doctor, Bruce underwent a stent placement, a surgical procedure to relieve the obstruction of the flow of bile. Within a week, his skin returned to normal and his pain was successfully relieved with smaller doses of medicine.

PALLIATIVE SURGERY

Surgery should be considered when there is a good chance that it will improve the patient's quality of life by reducing pain or decreasing the need for high doses of medication that cause unpleasant side effects. Palliative surgery may involve debulking (reducing the size of) a tumor that presses on nerves, or removal of organs that aggravate cancer symptoms. While results vary depending on the

Other Palliative Uses of Surgery

- Unblock the intestines.
- Unblock the bile ducts.
- Unblock the urinary system.
- Drain fluid that has built up in the abdomen (ascites).
- Gain access to an artery for injection of chemotherapy drugs.
- Remove or reduce the size of a pain-causing tumor that is unresponsive to other treatments.

type and size of the tumor and the procedure being performed, in some cases surgery may lead to longer-term symptom-free survival.

Surgery may also be performed to prevent further damage to the patient's body. For example, cancer that has spread to bones can weaken them, leading to fractures (breaks) that tend to heal very poorly. An operation to reinforce a bone with a metal rod can prevent some fractures and, if the bone is already broken, can rapidly relieve pain and help the patient return to routine activities. Surgical treatment of metastatic cancer near the spinal cord or large nerves can prevent or relieve symptoms such as paralysis and severe pain.

Nerve Blocks

Over the next several months, Bruce's pain became more intense, until his medication was again no longer adequate. A temporary nerve block to his celiac plexus (a group of nerves in the abdomen) provided good relief but lasted only a few weeks. Knowing that this technique had worked before, his doctor recommended a permanent block of his celiac plexus to relieve his abdominal pain. Although he experienced some temporary diarrhea, the nerve block provided Bruce with pain relief for months.

There are hundreds of nerves in the body that can be compressed by tumors. Compression can lead to pain in the areas of the body that a nerve goes through. This pain can be treated with temporary or permanent nerve blocks. A nerve block is a procedure in which medicines, sometimes combined with other chemicals, are injected into or around nerves, disrupting their ability to transmit pain signals. Depending on the location, extent, and severity of pain, nerve blocks may be directed at individual nerves, nerve bundles and nerve roots, or into the spaces that enclose the spinal cord.

One way to understand a nerve block is to imagine cutting an electrical wire to interrupt the flow of electricity. For example, pain in the chest or abdominal wall can be relieved by interrupting nerve signals that travel from these sites up through the spinal cord. A similar nerve blocking process can be performed to treat any of hundreds of nerves in the body. Pain in the legs, groin, and lower back can be relieved by injecting medicines into the epidural space surrounding the spinal column or directly into the intrathecal space where the spinal cord itself is located.

Nerve blocks can be performed on an outpatient basis or during surgery. There is no way to predict exactly how effective a nerve block will be because the amount of pain relief depends on the location of the pain, the type of medications used, and the individual patient response. Most people will experience at least some pain reduction from nerve blocks. However, patients with some types of pain may not benefit.

TEMPORARY NERVE BLOCKS

Temporary nerve blocks involve the injection of local anesthetics, such as lidocaine or bupivicaine, into or near nerves. Many people routinely undergo temporary nerve blocks when they receive a shot of novocaine at the dentist's office. Another commonly used temporary nerve block is epidural anesthesia during childbirth.

Pain relief from a temporary nerve block often occurs immediately, but may last only a few hours and need to be repeated frequently. Multiple injections may break a cycle of pain and inflammation, improve range of motion, and increase local blood flow. Doctors can repeat temporary nerve block injections as often as necessary because the procedure does not damage nerves. The addition of corticosteroid medicines (see Chapter 4) often extends the duration of pain relief to days or even weeks. Corticosteroids reduce swelling, irritation, and inflammation that occur when tumors press on nerves. Nerve blocks are used not only to relieve pain caused directly by cancer, but also to relieve secondary pain, such as that from muscle spasms, shingles, or nerve irritation.

Often, groups of nerves must be blocked simultaneously in order to achieve adequate pain relief. This may result in side effects in the area being treated such as muscle weakness, or abnormal tingling and burning sensations. Nerve blocks may also cause loss of sensation and even temporary paralysis in affected areas. If the area includes certain nerve groups in the abdomen, low blood pressure or temporary loss of bladder or bowel control may result.

Uses for Temporary Nerve Blocks

Temporary nerve blocks are performed for several reasons. A *therapeutic* nerve block, as described above, relieves pain. A *diagnostic* nerve block helps doctors to identify precisely which types of nerves are causing pain and guides decisions about pain treatment. A *prognostic* temporary nerve block may predict the outcome of long-lasting interventions, such as permanent nerve blocks or surgery, and may help determine if a patient is prone to side effects caused by nerve block medications. Unfortunately, the success of a temporary prognostic nerve block does not always mean more permanent approaches will work, but they do mimic the effects and provide doctors with clues about how to proceed with treatment. Sometimes a doctor will conduct a *preemptive* nerve block in advance of a procedure that is likely to have painful side effects in order to prevent pain from occurring.

PERMANENT NERVE BLOCKS

When temporary nerve blocks are insufficient to relieve pain or must be constantly repeated, a permanent nerve block may be performed. Permanent nerve blocks involve the injection of chemicals that destroy portions of a nerve, thus blocking pain signals for long periods of time, often many months. These blocks are not always "permanent" because many peripheral nerve cells (those outside of the brain or spinal cord) have the ability to regenerate over time.

Permanent nerve blocks are also called destructive blocks, neurolytic blockades, or neuroablation. They are usually reserved for patients who do not respond well to temporary nerve blocks or for patients whose cancer is not expected to get better. The best candidates for permanent nerve blocks are patients whose source of pain is easily identified and not widespread. Doctors usually prefer to avoid administering permanent nerve blocks when pain covers a wide area (an exception is abdominal pain) or is located in different parts of the body that are not close to one another.

The chemicals used to kill nerve cells include ethanol and phenol, and are called neurolytic agents, or simply neurolytics. An injection of ethanol can be extremely painful for a short time and must be accompanied by a local anesthetic. Phenol has anesthetic properties of its own and causes no pain when injected.

Permanent nerve blocks require the skill of doctors who specialize in anesthesiology. Destroying precisely the right nerves or nerve bundles that are responsible for the pain requires a great deal of skill. Neurolytic chemicals kill nerves indiscriminately, harming any with which they come into contact. For that reason, a prognostic temporary nerve block is usually done first to determine precisely where to inject nerve-destroying chemicals. Even after a permanent nerve block is done, opioids at lower doses are often prescribed to help control any remaining pain.

Though the most commonly used method to kill nerves is to inject them with neurolytics, other options are available. During radiofrequency ablation, a special probe is heated to very high temperatures and then applied to nerve cells. Cryoanalgesia is another option, which involves the use of an extremely cold probe that freezes and kills nerves.

SIDE EFFECTS OF NERVE BLOCKS

Side effects of temporary nerve blocks are usually limited and typically include muscle weakness and loss of sensation, both of which wear off as the medicines are flushed from the body. But the side effects associated with permanent nerve blocks may be serious and irreversible and can include muscle weakness, numbness, paralysis, and incontinence, depending on which nerves are harmed by neurolytic chemicals. The closer that nerve-killing agents are to the spinal cord, the more widespread side effects tend to be. Depending on where the nerves are located, the effects and side effects of nerve blocks differ.

LOCATION OF NERVE BLOCKS

Peripheral Nerve Blocks

Peripheral nerve blocks are most often used to treat pain in the head, chest, or abdomen. Peripheral nerves often overlap, requiring that more than one be blocked to relieve pain. These nerves transmit not only pain signals, but also information necessary for sensation and movement. When anesthetics are injected into peripheral nerves, they may interfere with these other activities and cause side effects, such as numbness or limited range of motion. Because of their potential for causing more serious side effects, permanent nerve block procedures are performed very cautiously and should be preceded by diagnostic nerve blocks to gauge the possible effects of more permanent options.

Central Nerve Blocks

Central nerve blocks involve injections of anesthetics or neurolytic agents into the epidural space that surrounds the spinal cord, or directly into the intrathecal space that houses the spinal cord itself (see Chapter 4, page 84). Temporary nerve blocks of this sort are regularly performed in hospitals to relieve back and neck pain and for women in labor. For some patients whose pain is hard to control, a permanent or semi-permanent catheter (drug delivery tube) can be inserted between the vertebrae (bones of the spine) and into the epidural or intrathecal spaces. Doctors, nurses, or other caregivers can inject anesthetics as needed, or the medicines can be delivered automatically by special pumps. Because chemicals are injected close to nerve roots, very small amounts of anesthetics or neurolytic agents can produce profound pain relief. Even opioids such as morphine can be injected directly into nerves in or around the spinal cord.

Central nerve blocks are usually performed by specially trained anesthesiologists. Permanent central nerve blocks are even more complicated and require the expertise of other specialists. The procedures are safest when performed in the mid-back and riskier with more chance of side effects when performed in the neck and lower back.

Permanent nerve blocks performed in and around the spine carry many potential risks, including partial or total paralysis, loss of sensation, incontinence, and, rarely, cardiac or respiratory depression.

Sympathetic Nerve Blocks

Sympathetic nerves connect the central nervous system to internal organs. Sympathetic nerve blocks can be used to relieve pain in patients with pancreatic cancer and other tumors that cause abdominal and back pain. They can also be used to treat pain in the arms or legs that is unresponsive to other therapies. These nerve blocks can lead to several side effects, such as temporary low blood pressure, diarrhea, urinary difficulties, and weakness in the lower extremities.

Spinal Opioid Infusion

For patients who require repeated temporary blocks or whose pain is difficult to control, an alternative to a permanent nerve block may be an infusion catheter implanted intraspinally, meaning into the area of the spinal cord. Catheter implantation is a relatively pain-free and quick procedure. The catheter allows doctors to give strong analgesics such as morphine and fentanyl (see Chapter 4) directly to nerves that cause pain. Medicines can be introduced as needed through the catheter with a syringe or automatically by an external infusion pump. In rare cases, tiny infusion pumps are surgically implanted inside the body, usually in the abdomen. These devices hold anesthetic reservoirs that last up to two months before a refill is required, but they are very expensive.

Because analgesic medicines are injected so close to the nerves, only small amounts are needed to produce significant, though temporary, pain relief. For example, patients who take morphine by mouth may need 100 to 1,000 mg per dose, compared with 1 to 10 mg when the drug flows through a spinal catheter. As with oral medications, patients may develop tolerance to intraspinal opioids and require higher doses to establish adequate pain control.

A home care nurse is usually needed to monitor treatment and teach patients and family members how to use and maintain infusion pumps and catheters. Unlike the effects of permanent nerve blocks, those of intraspinal opioid treatment are temporary and reversible.

Continuous opioid infusion is relatively safe and has few unwanted effects, but the technique is reserved for patients in whom oral medications do not provide enough relief or cause too many side effects. A potential complication is infection at the site of the catheter implant, which can become serious because it lies so close to the spine. Intraspinal opioids may also cause leg weakness and bladder incontinence.

Neurosurgery

Neurosurgery (nerve surgery) for pain control involves surgically cutting or destroying nerves that transmit pain signals. It is reserved as a last resort when other methods of pain control, including drug therapy and chemical nerve blocks, fail to provide sufficient relief. Because of the complexity, risks, and high costs, neurosurgery to relieve pain is rarely performed. These procedures must be performed by specialists called neurosurgeons at highly equipped treatment centers, and are therefore very expensive. Only patients with clearly localized pain are likely to benefit. Nerve surgery is irreversible and involves serious risks, including the temporary or permanent loss of feeling or motor control in some parts of the body, impaired reflexes, inability to distinguish temperature changes, and incontinence.

Cordotomy is the most frequently performed nerve surgery to relieve pain. During the operation, the surgeon cuts nerves in the spinal cord with a scalpel or destroys them with a very hot electrode. Cordotomies are used to relieve leg or hip pain on one side of the body. The technique is usually not helpful for patients with pain in the upper body. Nine out of ten people who undergo a cordotomy report significant pain relief, but the pain returns within a year for about half of the patients. Potential complications of the procedure include mild paralysis, loss of coordination, and most seriously, breathing difficulties.

Other pain relieving nerve surgeries include, rhizotomy, during which a surgeon cuts nerves coming out of the spinal cord, and neurectomy, which is used to treat nerves on the surface of the body.

Removal of the Pituitary Gland

The pituitary gland, a small gland located at the base of the brain, regulates the production of hormones. Hormones heavily influence some types of tumors and pain syndromes, so destroying or removing the pituitary (pituitary ablation) can reduce hormonal effects and decrease pain levels. After the doctor gives an anesthetic injection, a needle is inserted into the pituitary gland and a few drops of alcohol are injected, which kills the cells in the gland. Another option is to surgically remove the gland.

Removal of the pituitary gland is reserved for situations involving diffuse pain when other attempts at pain relief have failed and when regional pain control is not an option. Though the procedure may produce significant relief, particularly for patients with metastatic bone cancer, it is rarely performed. The operation can cause numerous side effects (including diabetes) and its benefits may last only a few months.

CHAPTER 6

Managing
Side Effects

Many patients believe the side effects of cancer treatment are worse than the treatment itself. But Tom's pain was so severe that he was willing to forego the side effects for relief of his pain. He did experience constipation initially, but after his first episode, his anticonstipation treatment was regulated so that he had no more trouble with constipation. He was also sleepy, but when his nurse explained to him that this would pass in a few days, he was willing to accept the sleepiness. And it did pass. Within five days of starting his pain medicine, which was adjusted daily, Tom was free of pain at last.

Cancer, cancer treatment, and analgesics for pain can cause various effects on the body. These side effects vary depending on the cause, and can range from mild to severe. Many of these side effects can be treated effectively or can be prevented. The success to effective management of side effects is an open and ongoing dialogue with your doctor and nurse.

Opioid Analgesic Side Effects

Opioid analgesics are often extremely effective in controlling cancer-related pain and discomfort, allowing you to conduct daily routines and participate in enjoyable activities in relative comfort. Yet the analgesics to control pain can cause side effects, some mild and others more serious. These may include constipation, nausea, vomiting, breathing difficulties, sedation, confusion, and delirium. In many cases, opioid-related side effects will ease or disappear after a few days as your body adjusts to the analgesics. But in some cases, the side effects may require medical attention.

There are many things that can be done to manage the side effects of opioid analgesics. In almost all cases, your doctor or nurse has many options to counteract and even completely eliminate them. Some measures may be started at the time of starting opioids to prevent side effects from occurring. While receiving opioid analgesics, communicate frequently with your health care team. As soon as you suspect that you are experiencing side effects, let your doctor or nurse know and ask for help. Members of your health care team can provide assistance when they are aware of your discomfort. It is essential to keep your doctor and nurses aware of your condition.

DIGESTIVE TRACT SIDE EFFECTS

Constipation

Constipation is the most common side effect among people who take opioids. The likelihood is so great that most doctors will prescribe a treatment to prevent the constipation. Even patients taking the weak opioids can develop constipation. The severity of constipation can range from mild to severe. It can cause decreased appetite, bloating, and abdominal cramps. If left untreated, constipation can become a source of pain and discomfort, and can lead to serious complications. In rare instances, constipation can be life-threatening. Fortunately, constipation is usually easy to treat with simple measures.

Because constipation and other digestive functions are highly personal, many people are embarrassed to talk freely about them with caregivers or medical personnel. Constipation can be prevented and controlled, so it is very important for you to discuss the problem openly and honestly in order to get treatment and relief from a condition that is not only uncomfortable, but potentially dangerous.

CAUSES OF CONSTIPATION

Opioid pain medication, taken orally or by injection, is the most common cause of constipation among people with cancer. Opioids cause waste products to move more slowly along the intestinal tract, allowing more time for water to be absorbed by the intestines. The result is stool that becomes hard and difficult

Notify Your Doctor or Nurse if:

- You cannot move your bowels within one or two days after taking a laxative.
- You have side effects of medication or other symptoms, such as persistent cramps, nausea, or vomiting.
- Your normal routine was one bowel movement a day and you haven't had one for three or four days, OR your normal routine was once every other day and you haven't had a bowel movement in four or five days.
- You experience severe straining on the toilet or commode.
- You experience severe abdominal pain or your abdomen feels harder than normal and very full, OR you notice red blood around the outside of the stools or have problems with hemorrhoids.
- You notice blood in or around the anal area or in stool.
- Constipation interferes with normal activities, such as walking or eating. How much constipation hinders your daily life is important to report because it indicates how severe the problem is and how quickly treatment should begin or if it should be increased.

When reporting your condition to your doctor or nurse, report all symptoms plus your bowel pattern and the day and type of the last movement. For example, if the doctor or nurse knows there are stains of stool on your clothes or your rectal area feels full, they know the lower bowel needs to be evacuated and a laxative is required.

to pass. As the dose of opioids increases, constipation may increase. The constipation may not diminish over time unless some measures are taken to treat it.

Some patients stop taking opioids without telling their doctors because constipation becomes so severe. This is not recommended since it will allow your pain to return. A better strategy is to inform your doctor or another member of your health care team about your condition so they can take steps to relieve both pain and constipation.

Factors that contribute to constipation include:

- lack of activity
- general weakness
- ignoring the urge to have a bowel movement
- inadequate fluid intake
- changes in diet or a diet that contains too little fiber
- emotional stress, anxiety, or depression
- dehydration caused by fever and vomiting
- other medicines, such as chemotherapy drugs

MANAGING CONSTIPATION

People with cancer should avoid treating constipation themselves without first seeking medical guidance. In most cases, constipation can be controlled with laxatives and dietary changes. Mild laxatives contain naturally occurring bulk fiber, which causes stool to retain water and stimulates the bowels to move waste products more quickly toward the rectum. Stool softeners are often prescribed along with laxatives to draw moisture into the bowel, allowing stool to move more easily through the digestive tract. Commonly used mild laxatives include Doxidan and Senokot. Laxatives combined with a stool softener include Senokot-S, casanthranol with Colace (Peri-Colace).

Patients who take opioid medicines usually begin an anticonstipation bowel program at the same time they start their opioid analgesics to prevent or at least minimize constipation. Patients with kidney disease should avoid laxatives containing magnesium, and those with heart disease should avoid laxatives that contain sodium.

Once constipation begins, stool softeners alone are rarely enough to relieve constipation. Doctors often prescribe laxatives and stool softeners together for the best results. You should consult with your doctor before using any of these products to determine how much and how often you should take them. Doses of these medications should be gradually increased until they become effective.

Sometimes, stronger laxatives, such as magnesium hydroxide (Milk of Magnesia) and magnesium citrate are needed to stimulate the bowels. The level of medication should be enough to help the patient produce bowel movements regularly—usually no more than two days apart.

High Fiber Foods

Breads and Cereals	Serving Size	Dietary Fiber (grams)
Bran cereals	1/2 cup	3–13
Popcorn	2 cups	5
Brown rice	1/2 cup	6
Whole-wheat bread	1 slice	1–2
Wheat bran, raw	1/4 cup	6
Legumes		
Kidney beans*	1/2 cup	8
Navy beans*	1/2 cup	9
Vegetables		
Broccoli*	1/2 cup	4
Brussel sprouts*	1/2 cup	3
Carrots	1/2 cup	2
Corn	1/2 cup	5
Green peas	1/2 cup	3
Potato with skin	1 medium	3
Fruit		
Apple with peel	1 medium	4
Banana	1 medium	2
Blueberries	1/2 cup	2
Pear with skin	1 medium	5
Prunes	3	3
Orange	1 medium	3
Raisins	1/4 cup	3
Strawberries	1 cup	3

* These foods tend to cause gas.

Source: Oncology Nutrition Patient Education Materials. ©1998 American Dietetic Association.
Used by permission.

Adequate fluid intake is just as important as the use of laxatives. Doctors recommend eight to ten glasses of liquid daily, including water and fruit juices. Another remedy is to eat foods that contain high amounts of fiber (see page 117). The recommended intake of fiber is 25 to 35 grams a day. Exercise is also an important component of preventing constipation, if appropriate in your situation.

When constipation becomes severe and doesn't respond to laxatives and dietary adjustments, doctors may take more aggressive measures, such as suppositories or enemas, which may be appropriate for patients who are unable to keep food down and therefore cannot ingest adequate amounts of fiber through diet or laxatives. One option is a suppository inserted into the rectum to stimulate the lower bowel. Suppositories should not be used for cancer patients who have low platelet or white blood cell counts because the suppository capsule may break small blood vessels in the rectal area, creating a risk of bleeding or infection.

The last alternative for patients with severe constipation is an enema, which often brings immediate relief while causing minimal discomfort. Only one or two enemas are usually needed to relieve even severe constipation. Enema kits and commercial enema preparations, such as Fleet's, can be purchased at pharmacies without a prescription. Enema solutions containing mixtures of water and mineral oil or soap suds can be made at home. It is best to give an enema lying on your left side near a bathroom or with a portable commode next to the bed or couch. Before performing an enema at home, always check with a doctor or nurse. People who have lower colon surgery or other conditions involving the lower colon and rectum might not be able to have an enema.

Fecal Impaction

Constipation that persists because of insufficient treatment or poor patient compliance with medical instructions can lead to a condition called fecal impaction. This occurs when pieces of dried stool become lodged in the rectum or intestines and block the ability of the gastrointestinal system to empty. Left untreated, fecal impaction can be dangerous. If it is not diagnosed and patients continue to take strong laxatives, the bowel may rupture behind the impaction. Most fecal impactions occur in the rectum. The most common treatment is for the doctor or nurse to manually remove the stool with a gloved finger, then wash the area with an enema. The procedure may be painful and require an anesthetic or sedative for comfort. Fecal impaction that occurs higher in the colon can usually be eliminated with enemas.

Tips for Preventing and Managing Constipation

The best way to manage constipation is to prevent it. Patients can take the following steps to minimize the risk of developing constipation when taking opioid medications:

- Drinking lots of fluids is the most important action you can take. Drink eight to ten cups of liquid each day (if allowed by your doctor). Try water, prune juice, warm juices, teas, and hot lemonade.
- Try to eat at the same times each day.
- Avoid liquids that contain caffeine.
- Eat foods high in fiber, such as uncooked fruits (with the skin on), vegetables, whole grain breads and cereals, fresh raw fruits with skins and seeds, dates, apricots, prunes, and nuts.
- Add one or two tablespoons of unprocessed bran to your food. This adds bulk and stimulates bowel movements. Keep a shaker of bran handy at mealtimes to make it easy to sprinkle on foods.
- Avoid foods and beverages that cause gas such as cabbage, broccoli, cauliflower, cucumbers, dried beans, peas, onions, and carbonated drinks.
- Get as much exercise as you can, even if it means just walking a short distance.
- Try to have a bowel movement whenever you have the urge.
- Use stool softeners or laxatives only as instructed by your doctor or nurse.
- Use a rectal suppository only after checking with your doctor or nurse.
- If you are confined to bed, try to use the toilet or bedside commode when you have a bowel movement, even if that is the only time you get out of bed.
- Use an enema to provide immediate relief from constipation, but first check with the doctor or nurse. Enemas should be the last step for relieving constipation. They evacuate the lower bowel and help the upper bowel move as well.

Do Not:
- Strain or use extreme force when trying to move your bowels.
- Use over-the-counter laxatives or enemas unless discussed with your doctor.
- Eat foods that can cause constipation, such as chocolate, cheese, eggs, and refined grain products (cakes, cookies, donuts, etc.).
- Use laxatives and enemas if you have a low white blood count or low platelet count.

Elderly patients, especially those who are easily confused, may not know that they have fecal impaction because at first the condition may cause no symptoms except lack of bowel movements. Instead, patients complain of pressure in the abdomen caused by the blockage. Diarrhea may even occur, as loose stool and mucus seeps around the blockage and leaks from the rectum. This can cause skin breakdown, infections of the urinary tract, total bowel obstruction, and bacterial infection from the intestines.

Nausea and Vomiting

Nausea is an extremely unpleasant condition that can cause minimal difficulties to a great deal of suffering. It can leave people weak and unable to carry out normal routines. People with severe nausea often find that they cannot even get out of bed. Vomiting often accompanies nausea, but not always.

Frequent nausea and vomiting can also lead to serious complications, such as dehydration or aspirating (breathing in) food or liquids. In addition, people suffering from nausea typically have no desire to eat, which further weakens them.

CAUSES OF NAUSEA AND VOMITING

Opioids produce nausea and vomiting by stimulating the vomiting center in the brain and they have effects on the gastrointestinal (GI) tract. Approximately one-third of all patients who take opioids will experience some degree of nausea. However, the body usually becomes tolerant to opioid-caused nausea after a few days and the side effects disappear. Constipation, which is almost always a side effect of opioids, can also lead to nausea.

Sometimes patients who experience nausea when first starting their opioid medication think they are "allergic" to the medicine. Nausea is not a sign of an allergy, and patients should be warned when first starting the medication that nausea is a common side effect.

Nonsteroidal anti-inflammatory drugs (NSAIDs) can also cause nausea and vomiting in some patients. When taken for a long period of time, NSAIDs irritate the stomach lining and can also cause ulcer-like symptoms. Other sources of cancer-related nausea include tumors that partially or completely block the intestinal tract, and injury to abdominal tissue and kidneys from radiation therapy. Nausea may also result from tumors in the brain or those that have spread from their original site to other parts of the body

Notify Your Doctor or Nurse if:

- You experience unrelieved nausea or vomiting.
- You vomit more than three times an hour for three or more hours.
- You cannot take in more than four cups of liquid or ice chips in a day or cannot eat for more than two days.
- You cannot take medications because of nausea or vomiting.
- You feel weak and dizzy.

The following could be related to other causes of nausea and vomiting but still need to be reported to your doctor:

- You notice blood or material that looks like coffee grounds in your vomit. (This could signal bleeding inside the gastrointestinal tract.)
- Vomit shoots straight out for a distance (projectile vomiting). This may mean that there are problems in the stomach or intestine that should be investigated by the doctor.
- You experience severe stomach pain while vomiting.

(metastatic tumors). Nausea and vomiting are also two of the most common side effects of chemotherapy.

MANAGING NAUSEA AND VOMITING

The good news is that nausea and vomiting related to opioid analgesics can almost always be relieved with medications called antiemetics. Fortunately, doctors have a number of antiemetics at their disposal. Different antiemetics work for different people, and it may be necessary to try more than one before you get relief. Continue to work with your doctor and nurse to find the medicine that works best for you.

When starting opioid analgesics, patients should be told that nausea can be a side effect and that it is usually short-lived and controllable. Routine preventive use of antinausea medicines may not be necessary, but patients should have access to these medicines in case they are needed. Usually, when first starting

(continued on page 124)

Tips for Managing Nausea

- Be sure that your doctor or nurse is aware of your nausea.
- Use antiemetics (antinausea medicine) as instructed by your doctor or nurse.
- Stay in bed for an hour or so after receiving pain medication to reduce the risk of nausea. (Moving around after treatment increases the likelihood of feeling ill.)
- If nausea occurs only between meals, eat frequent, small meals and snacks at bedtime.
- Avoid fried foods, dairy products, and acidic foods such as fruit juices or vinegar salad dressing. Fried and acidic foods are hard to digest and may make nausea worse.
- Seek out the foods you like. Many people develop a distaste for red meat and meat broths. Exchange other protein sources such as fish and chicken.
- Eat foods with pleasant aromas, such as lemon drops or mints.
- Avoid unpleasant or strong odors. Eat food cold or at room temperature to decrease its smell and taste.
- Drink clear liquids served cold and sipped slowly (e.g., ginger ale, apple juice, broth, tea) or eat Popsicles or Jell-O.
- Chew gum, hard candy, or candied ginger. Candied ginger can help reduce nausea, but shouldn't be eaten in large quantities. Peppermint may also help.
- Allow fresh air into the house or go outside. Taking in more oxygen helps calm the stomach and decrease feelings of nausea.
- Rest. Some people find it helpful to lie down when they are nauseated.
- Drink fluids two hours after vomiting to replenish losses. Let the fizz go out of sodas before drinking them because carbonation can upset the stomach.
- Eat bland foods, such as dry toast and crackers.
- Try to rest quietly for at least an hour after each meal.
- Rinse out your mouth frequently. This not only removes unpleasant tastes that upset the stomach, but also protects teeth and soft tissue from corrosive stomach acids.
- Wear loosely fitting clothes. Tight-fitting material puts pressure on the throat and stomach.
- Distract attention by watching television, listening to music, reading, or visiting with company.
- When you begin to feel nauseated, relax and take slow deep breaths.

Tips for Managing Vomiting

What to Do:

- If you are in bed, lie on your side so that you won't inhale the material vomited.
- Request that medications be prescribed in suppository form.
- Take liquids in the form of ice chips or frozen juice chips that can be munched slowly.

Do Not:

- Force foods or fluids when nauseated or vomiting.
- Lie flat on your back.
- Eat foods that are sweet, fatty, salty, or spicy, or foods that have strong smells.
- Expose yourself to unnecessary stimulation or excitement.
- Eat anything for four to eight hours if you vomit often.
- Take only clear liquids for more than two days in a row.

Things to Discuss with Your Doctor or Nurse:

- How long has nausea been a problem?
- When did it begin and how long has it lasted?
- When does it occur in relation to taking your opioid analgesic?
- How bad was the most recent nausea?
- How much does the nausea interfere with normal activities?
- Was medicine prescribed for nausea or vomiting?
- Were any non-prescription medicines taken for the nausea?
- Was nausea followed by vomiting?
- What did the vomit look like? Was it the same color as earlier vomit?
- How often has vomiting happened in the last 24 hours?
- Is there anything that makes it better or worse?
- What other symptoms are new since the nausea or vomiting began?
- What and how much was eaten in the last 24 hours?
- What and how much liquid was taken in the last 24 hours?

opioids in patients who have not received them before, some of the milder antinausea medicines, such as prochlorperazine (Compazine) or metoclopramide (Reglan), are sufficient. If nausea continues with the milder antinausea medicines given as needed, then antinausea medicines should be given on a regular schedule. If nausea persists for more than one week, the doctor will usually reconsider the cause of the nausea. If the nausea is related to the opioid, then the doctor may:

- change the opioid to another opioid medicine
- add an adjuvant analgesic in order to reduce the dose of opioid
- give a stronger antinausea medicine such as granisetron (Kytril) or ondansetron (Zofran)

CENTRAL NERVOUS SYSTEM SIDE EFFECTS

Respiratory Depression

Respiratory depression is slow, shallow breathing. Many people think that this is a very common effect of opioids. Although it does not happen often, it causes patients and families a great deal of anxiety.

Notify Your Doctor or Nurse if:

- You experience slow breathing.
- Your skin looks pale or takes on a bluish color.
- Your skin feels cold and clammy.
- Your family cannot awaken you, or has difficulty arousing you.
- You have any confusion.

CAUSES OF RESPIRATORY DEPRESSION

Respiratory depression is related to the effect of the opioids on the central nervous system. Along with respiratory depression, confusion and sedation can also occur. In fact, if respiratory depression occurs, it is usually accompanied by sedation and mental clouding.

Respiratory depression rarely occurs, except in patients who have never had opioids before and those who may have significant lung disease. It is potentially the most serious of all the side effects related to opioid analgesics. But, it is a very unusual side effect of opioids that are given to treat cancer pain, as long as the opioid dose is appropriate to the degree of pain. It is also less likely to occur when patients have normal liver and kidney function.

With repeated opioid use, the risk of opioid-caused respiratory depression decreases over time. As a result, opioid analgesics can be used to treat cancer pain without significant risk of respiratory depression.

MANAGING RESPIRATORY DEPRESSION

Respiratory depression from opioid analgesics that does not resolve with continued use of opioids is usually controlled with the medication naloxone (Narcan) which temporarily blocks the action of opioids. If you are taking opioids for your pain, call your doctor immediately if you experience slow breathing (less than eight breaths per minute) or very shallow breathing (short breaths that don't take in much air).

Tips for Managing Respiratory Depression

- Remain calm.
- Do not stop your opioid medicines without first talking with your doctor.
- Do not increase your opioid therapy without your doctor's advice.
- Notify your doctor if you are taking any medicines that he or she might not know about (including herbs, vitamins, or any other supplements).

Sedation

Another side effect that occurs as a result of the effect of opioids on the central nervous system is sedation, or feeling drowsy. It is an important dose-limiting effect of opioid therapy, which means that it can lead patients to limit the amount of opioids they take even though their pain remains unrelieved. Patients should be forewarned about this effect.

CAUSES OF SEDATION

Starting opioid therapy or significantly increasing the dose of the opioid can cause sedation that can last until tolerance develops, usually with days to weeks. In some patients, what may look like sedation related to opioid therapy might actually be a natural effect of pain relief in someone who has been without sleep. Do not confuse this natural "catching" up of sleep with over-sedation. Other factors that can cause sedation include the use of other medicines that could cause sedation or other illnesses or disease.

MANAGING SEDATION

Usually the sedation will subside within a few to several days. If the sedation persists, it is usually best treated by reducing the opioid in each dose while increasing the dose frequency. In some patients, the doctor might switch to another opioid to reduce the effect of sedation. Giving long-acting or sustained-release opioids can decrease sedation. These medicines may not meet the patient's changing pain needs, so they might be combined with short-acting opioids that can be used as "rescue" therapy for breakthrough pain.

Notify Your Doctor or Nurse if:

- Sedation lasts more than one week.
- Your family cannot arouse you.
- You are concerned about the amount of time you are sleeping.
- Any confusion occurs.
- There is a decrease in your rate of breathing.

Tips for Managing Sedation

- It is often best to avoid driving for two weeks after starting opioids or increasing dose.
- Do not confuse "catching up" on sleep with sedation.
- Notify your doctor if you are taking any medicines that he or she might not know about (including herbs, vitamins, or any other supplements).

Confusion and Delirium

For patients and their families, confusion and delirium are frightening effects of opioids. Delirium is characterized by a change in mental function, a disturbance in level of consciousness with reduced ability to focus or shift attention, and disturbance that develops within a short time and fluctuates throughout the day. Symptoms include difficulty sleeping, nightmares, irritability, anxiety, difficulty concentrating, attention deficits, memory disturbances, and psychomotor behavior such as picking at bed covers.

Causes of Confusion and Delirium

This side effect results from the effect of the opioids on the central nervous system. With delirium, the first manifestation may be something as mild as nightmares but can progress rapidly to the patient developing something as severe as hallucinations. Mild brain function impairment is common after starting opioids or increasing a dose. However, major brain impairment is usually temporary in most patients, lasting from a few days to a week or two.

Persistent confusion due to opioid use alone can occur, but the cause of persistent confusion is usually related to a combined effect of the opioid and other factors. These factors can include fluid and electrolyte imbalances, tumor involvement of the brain or central nervous system, major organ problems, or reduced oxygen.

Notify Your Doctor or Nurse if:

- You are having any of the symptoms of delirium.
- You are confused.
- You are having any other symptoms.
- You are taking any medicines that your doctor might not know about (including herbs, vitamins, or any other supplements).
- You have a fever, chills, or other symptom of infection.

MANAGING DELIRIUM

The doctor will evaluate the cause of the delirium. The underlying cause of the delirium will be treated. If the cause is the opioid analgesic, for some patients, lowering the dose of the opioid can resolve the side effect. For others, the opioid may need to be changed. Other medicines that could be contributing to the delirium will be stopped and the recent cancer treatment will be reviewed. Many doctors will ask for an evaluation by a psychiatrist to be certain of the underlying cause. The patient should be surrounded by familiar people, objects, and sounds and aware of time, place, and date on a frequent basis.

Tips for Managing Delirium

- Surround yourself with familiar family, friends, objects, and sounds.
- Have a family member or friend stay with you if delirium occurs.
- Have someone orient you to time, place, and date several times each day.
- Have someone notify your doctor if symptoms increase or change.
- Notify your doctor if you are taking any medicines that he or she might not know about (including herbs, vitamins, or any other supplements).

Other Side Effects

Opioid medicines occasionally cause itching, which can be severe at times, but it usually decreases over time. Itching can also be caused by chemotherapy and radiation therapy as well as other medical conditions or other medicines. Dry skin can also lead to itching. It can irritate the skin tissues to the point of cracking open. Itching may contribute to increased restlessness, anxiety, skin sores (from scratching) and, in extreme cases, infection. Itching accompanied by a rash and other symptoms (such as difficulty breathing or swelling of the face) may indicate a medicine allergy. It is important for the doctor to identify the cause of the itching so appropriate treatment can be given.

Managing Itching and Other Skin Problems

Itching and other skin problems are not usually an emergency, but they can be upsetting and uncomfortable for the person who has them and can indicate other medical problems. After identifying the cause of the itching, your doctor may recommend some of the remedies below for minimizing itching caused by the condition. One of the main problems with itching is that skin will breakdown and can lead to infections.

Notify Your Doctor or Nurse if:

- Itching becomes severe or does not subside after two or more days.
- Your skin takes on a yellowish color or if your urine turns the color of tea.
- Your skin has open sores and looks red.
- A rash becomes worse after creams or ointments have been applied.
- Foul-smelling drainage from your skin develops.
- You become very anxious and restless (e.g., cannot sleep through the night due to itching).
- You develop hives, itching, or swelling of the face after taking pain medications.

Tips for Minimizing Itching
and Other Skin Problems

- Apply water-soluble skin creams such as aloe vera lotion two to three times a day, especially after a bath when the skin is damp.
- Limit bathing to once a day or less and use warm instead of hot water.
- Add baking soda, mineral oil, or bath oil to bath water.
- Wash skin gently using a mild soap and pat skin dry.
- Use baking soda instead of deodorant.
- Apply cool, wet packs (crushed ice in a plastic bag which is then wrapped in a towel) to the skin, remove it when it becomes warm, let skin dry; reapply as needed.
- Keep nails clean and cut short.
- Try rubbing, pressure, or vibration instead of scratching.
- Rub itchy areas with a cool cloth.
- Wear loose clothing made of a soft fabric.
- Change bed sheets daily.
- Keep rooms cool (60° to 70°F) and well ventilated.
- Drink as much water and other fluids as possible (at least eight glasses every day).
- Get adequate rest.
- Take medications for itching as ordered by doctor.
- Cover up in the sun and use a lotion with at least a #15 SPF.
- Use an electric razor rather than razor blades.

Do Not:
- Use hot water for baths.
- Scrub skin; instead, be gentle.
- Wear tight clothing.
- Use harsh detergents.
- Go outside in extremely hot, cold, or windy conditions.
- Wear colognes, after-shaves, or after-bath splashes that contain alcohol.
- Open or pop blisters.

Diarrhea, the passage of loose or watery stools, results when fluids in the intestines are not reabsorbed back into the body. Diarrhea can cause serious health consequences, such as dehydration, weakness, and anxiety. It can also lead to rectal infection because the acids and irritants in the diarrhea stool can cause the skin to break, which allows bacteria to invade the body. Because of the problems that may arise, diarrhea should be treated as soon as possible.

Causes of Diarrhea

One of the primary causes of diarrhea among patients with cancer pain is the overuse of laxatives to combat constipation from opioid medications. Diarrhea can also be a side effect of chemotherapy and radiation therapy given to the abdomen. Other causes include infections, surgery, lactose intolerance (inability to digest milk products), anxiety, and supplemental feedings containing large amounts of vitamins, minerals, sugar, and electrolytes.

Managing Diarrhea

Taking antidiarrhea medicines is the fastest way to stop diarrhea. These medicines slow down the actions of the bowel and allow more time for the intestines to absorb water. Over-the-counter antidiarrheals include Kaopectate and Pepto-Bismol. For more severe cases, your doctor may prescribe Lomotil or paregoric.

Changing your diet is often a very effective remedy. Avoid foods that increase the action of the bowel and decrease its ability to pull fluids out of stool. Avoid products that contain caffeine or produce gas. Low-fat, low-fiber foods are better choices (see below). Nutmeg is also believed by some to help slow down the gastrointestinal tract. Patients with chronic diarrhea should drink water to replace fluid losses caused by diarrhea.

The lower abdomen can become quite sore from intestinal cramps that may accompany diarrhea. Diarrhea can also cause fatigue. Rectal skin or skin around a stoma (an opening in the skin on the abdomen for stool to come out into a bag) can become very sore. There are several ways to ease abdominal or skin soreness and increase comfort:

1. Put a warm water bottle wrapped in a towel on the abdomen. Warmth on the stomach can relieve pain and discomfort caused by stomach tightness or

Notify Your Doctor or Nurse if:

- You have severe diarrhea.
- You experience diarrhea for more than one day.
- You notice blood in the diarrhea stool.
- You get a fever above 100.5°F with diarrhea.
- You have six to eight or more loose bowel movements per day with no improvement after two days.
- When taking pain medicines you are unable to hold in stool when this was not a problem before.
- You notice blood in or around the anal area or in stool.
- You lose five pounds after diarrhea starts.
- You have new abdominal cramps or pain for two days or more.
- You do not urinate for twelve hours or more.
- You do not drink any liquids for more than two days.
- You cannot maintain adequate fluid intake.
- Your abdomen suddenly becomes puffy or bloated.
- You have been constipated for several days and begin to experience a small amount of diarrhea or oozing of fecal material. This suggests an impaction.
- You experience other symptoms with the diarrhea, such as stomach pain, stomach cramps, bloating, nausea, vomiting, fever, or bloody stool.

Things to Discuss with Your Doctor or Nurse:
- How many bowel movements are usual each day?
- How many bowel movements have there been in the last twenty-four hours?
- How runny were they?
- Have you been taking your pain medicines as directed?
- How much liquid was taken and how much food was eaten in the last two days? This information helps the doctor or nurse know if your body is receiving enough to replace what is being lost. Sometimes intravenous (IV) fluids are ordered to balance the fluid loss and replace water, vitamins, and minerals.
- What other medicines were taken in the last two or three days (chemotherapy, laxatives, antidiarrhea tablets or liquids, non-prescription and herbal medicines)?
- Have you lost weight? How much?
- Is there any history of other bowel problems, such as diverticulitis, colitis, or irritable bowel syndrome?

Changing Your Diet
Can Help Control Diarrhea

Foods to Choose
- cottage cheese and other low-fat cheeses
- eggs (not fried)
- yogurt
- broth
- poultry
- ground beef
- fish (not fried)
- applesauce
- apples without skins
- apple or grape juice
- white bread or toast
- rice pudding
- custard
- tapioca made with low-fat milk
- gelatin
- hot cooked cereals
- white pasta or rice
- potatoes
- cooked vegetables such as green beans, carrots, peas, spinach or squash, or soups made from these vegetables

Foods to Avoid
- fried or greasy foods
- raw fruits and vegetables
- pastries
- potato chips
- pretzels
- strong spices
- olives
- pickles
- beans
- broccoli
- onions
- cabbage

cramps. However, do not use a heating pad or very hot water in the water bottle. The skin may be overly sensitive to heat, especially if you are receiving chemotherapy or radiation therapy.

2. After a bout of diarrhea, cleanse the outside of the rectum gently with warm water and then dry the skin to reduce redness and prevent infection.

3. Soak in warm water. Use a tub or Sitz bath. Sitz baths are plastic bowls that are placed over the toilet; you can sit in the bowl of warm water while it spills into the toilet below. Sitting in a bathtub of warm water can also be helpful.

4. Apply soothing creams, ointments, or astringent pads such as Tucks to the rectal area. Creams prevent rectal skin from chapping in the same way they

Tips for Managing Diarrhea

- Try a clear liquid diet (water, weak tea, apple juice, peach nectar, clear broth, popsicles, plain gelatin) as soon as diarrhea starts or when you feel that it's going to start.
- Drink at least eight to ten glasses of water a day to prevent dehydration.
- Eat frequent small meals.
- When the diarrhea starts to improve, try eating small amounts of low-fiber foods such as rice, bananas, applesauce, yogurt, mashed potatoes, low-fat cottage cheese, and dry toast.
- If diarrhea lasts longer than two days, start a liquid diet and add low-fiber foods as tolerated.
- Monitor amount and frequency of bowel movements.
- Clean the anal area with a mild soap after each bowel movement; rinse well with warm water and pat dry.
- Inspect the anal area for red, scaly, broken skin. If present, notify your doctor or nurse.
- Apply a water-repellent cream such as A & D ointment to the anal area; the doctor may prescribe a local anesthetic ointment as well.
- Sitz baths may help reduce discomfort.
- Take medicine for diarrhea as ordered by your doctor.

prevent diaper rash or chapping on infants' skin. Try Nupercainal, A & D ointment, or Vaseline.

5. If diarrhea continues and the rectal area becomes very sore and red, apply an ointment such as Desitin to protect the skin.

6. Protect the bed and chairs from being soiled by putting two overlapping waterproof pads or Chux (also called blue pads) under the buttocks where you lay or sit.

SEXUALITY ISSUES

People undergoing cancer therapy may experience greatly decreased levels of sexual desire. Causes include pain and pain treatment, side effects of treatment,

- Fatigue accompanying diarrhea may indicate low potassium levels. Increase potassium intake by eating foods that contain high levels of this important mineral (e.g., bananas, potatoes, apricots, green beans, halibut, and asparagus tips) or by taking potassium supplements. Check with your doctor first.

Do Not:
- Eat foods that may stimulate or irritate the digestive tract such as: high fiber foods such as whole grain breads and cereal; products with bran; fried or greasy foods; nuts, raw fruits, or vegetables; rich pastries, candy, jellies; strong spices and herbs.
- Drink caffeinated, alcoholic, or carbonated beverages and do not use tobacco products.
- Consume milk and milk products, such as creamed soups, puddings, or milk shakes.
- Do not eat very hot or very cold foods.
- Do not take only clear liquids for more than two days in a row.

or depression. Sex is a very sensitive subject and coping with sexual problems requires careful thought and planning of both partners.

Try to keep an open mind about ways to feel sexual pleasure. Some couples have a narrow idea of what is "normal" in sex. If both partners cannot reach orgasm through or during penetration, they feel cheated. For people who are experiencing cancer pain, however, there may be times when intercourse is not possible.

Those times can be opportunities to learn new ways to give and receive sexual pleasure. At times, just cuddling can be pleasure enough. Do not deny yourself other ways of showing caring and feeling alive, just because your "normal" routine has been disrupted.

Notify Your Doctor or Nurse if:

- You experience pain during intercourse.
- You have questions about when to have intercourse.
- Your sexual partner is fearful.
- You are concerned about having little or no interest in sexual activities or feelings.
- You have concerns about pregnancy.

Gather as many facts as you can about the usual effects of your cancer, pain, or pain treatment on sexuality. Talk with your doctor, nurse, or any other member of your health care team. When you know what to expect, you can plan ways to handle those issues. Strive for good communication about sex with your partner and with your doctor. Good communication is also the key to changing your sexual routine when you have cancer pain. If some part of your body is tender or sore, let your partner know.

Managing Pain Related to Sexual Activity for Women

The physical effects of medications and treatment, including nausea, constipation, and fatigue, may leave little energy for intimacy. But, sexual desire often returns as side effects diminish. Pain during intercourse is a common problem for female cancer patients. The pain is often related to changes in the vagina's size or moistness, which can occur after pelvic surgery, radiation therapy, or treatment that affects a woman's hormones. If you don't produce enough natural lubrication in your vagina, intercourse can be dry and painful and can leave a burning feeling or soreness. The risk of repeated urinary tract infections or irritation also increases. Some cancer treatments cause genital pain. Others, such as radiation therapy, may change the size and shape of the vagina, causing it to become shorter and narrower, which results in painful intercourse.

Sometimes the pain sets off a problem called vaginismus, in which the muscles around the opening of the vagina become tense without the woman's awareness. Her partner's penis cannot enter the vagina, and if he pushes harder, the woman's pain becomes greater because her vaginal muscles are clenched in spasm. Vaginismus can be treated with counseling and some special relaxation training.

Tips for Women to Minimize Pain and Improve Sexual Pleasure

- Plan sexual activity for the time of day when your pain is weakest. If you are using pain medication, take it at an hour before so that it will be in full effect during sex. Try to find doses of medication somewhere between total pain relief and getting too drowsy.
- Focus on your feelings of pleasure and excitement, letting any painful feelings slip into the background.
- Make sure you feel very aroused before you start intercourse. It is only when you are highly excited that your vagina expands and the walls of your vagina produce lubricating fluid. As women go through menopause, whether as a result of aging or because of cancer treatment, it may take a longer time and more touching to get fully aroused.
- Spread a large amount of water-based lubricating gel in and around your vagina before having intercourse. You can also use lubrication suppositories before intercourse or a vaginal moisturizer that you apply a few times each week.
- Empty your bladder before intercourse or before touching.
- Let your partner know if any kind of touching causes pain. Show him ways to caress you or positions that aren't painful.
- Find a position for touching or intercourse that puts as little pressure as possible on the painful areas of your body. If it helps, support the painful area of your body and limit its movement with pillows. If a certain motion is painful, choose a position that doesn't require it.

Even pain in a nongenital part of the body can interfere with a woman's pleasure during sex. For example, pain such as arm soreness after a radical mastectomy or tingling in the hands and feet after some types of chemotherapy may be enough to reduce sexual desire or enjoyment. Pain may even make it hard for a woman to use intercourse positions that worked well in the past.

Tips for Men to Minimize Pain and Improve Sexual Pleasure

- Learn what changes to expect and how long they will last if you are taking hormone medications as a cancer treatment. In some cases, the level of testosterone falls after certain treatments. A low testosterone level can cause problems with erections and even lower sexual desire. The doctor can check testosterone blood levels, and in some cases can prescribe additional testosterone medication doses if the levels are too low.
- Ask if "dry" orgasms will happen. When a man has the feeling of an orgasm, but does not ejaculate, it is called a "dry orgasm." Certain treatments cause more sex-related nerve and blood vessel damage than others. Nerve and blood vessel injury near the penis or prostate, or in the pelvic area, changes the way men experience desire, erections, and orgasms. They can also affect whether men continue to ejaculate.
- Ask about penile implants and other options if erections are a problem. Surgeons and urologists know about the options and can discuss the pros and cons of each.
- Keep in mind that you will almost always be able to be intimate and feel pleasure from touching. For example, some types of treatment can damage a man's ability to have erections. Few cancer treatments (other than those affecting some areas of the brain or spinal cord) damage the nerves and muscles involved in feeling pleasure from touch and reaching orgasm. Most men who cannot have erections or produce semen can still have the feeling of orgasm with the right kind of touching. Pleasure and satisfaction are possible, even if some aspects of sexuality have changed. The best time to try to be intimate is when the cancer pain is controlled.

Managing Pain Related to Sexual Activity for Men

Men also sometimes feel genital pain during sex. Irritation of the prostate gland or urethra from cancer treatment can cause painful ejaculation. Cancer treatments or cancer pain can also interfere with erections or cause premature ejaculation (reaching a climax too quickly). Medical or surgical procedures can often restore erections, and premature ejaculation can be overcome with some practice in slowing down excitement (see *Additional Reading* listed in the Resources section for more information).

Tiredness and fatigue (lack of energy) are common side effects associated with cancer, treatment, and pain. Fatigue can occur suddenly and can be overwhelming. It is not always relieved by rest, and it can last well after treatment ends. Treatment-related fatigue affects many aspects of a person's life, including the ability to conduct normal activities.

Notify Your Doctor or Nurse if:

- You have trouble waking up, even after others try to rouse you.
- You feel like you have no energy.
- You sleep more than usual.
- You do not want to do normal activities.
- Your attention to personal appearance decreases.
- You feel tired even after sleeping.
- You feel confused or have trouble concentrating.
- You are too tired to get out of bed for more than a twenty-four hour period.
- You feel confused.
- Fatigue becomes progressively worse.
- You experience frequent dizziness or loss of balance when getting out of bed or moving from a sitting to a standing position.

Causes of Tiredness and Fatigue

Many factors can cause these symptoms, and it can sometimes be difficult to determine the exact cause. Opioids can cause tiredness in many people, but it usually diminishes after a few days. Patients may feel tired because their normal rest and sleep habits are disrupted or because they feel depressed or are in pain. Other sources of tiredness and fatigue include chemotherapy or radiation therapy, poor nutrition, anemia, infection, the effects of chemicals produced by tumors, and an imbalance of chemicals in the body called electrolytes.

Managing Tiredness and Fatigue

People with cancer often say they feel more tired than ever before in their lives. Tiredness and fatigue may be unavoidable consequences of cancer, treatment, and pain. But, there are some things you can do to reduce the tiredness and make the best use of the energy that you have.

Tips for Managing Tiredness and Fatigue

- Plan rest periods to conserve energy for important things.
- Plan your day's activities so you are with people or on trips when you feel the most refreshed and awake.
- Schedule necessary activities throughout the day rather than all at once; light activity may be helpful.
- Get enough rest and sleep.
- Eat a nutritious diet and drink plenty of liquids.
- Let others help you with meals, housework, or errands.
- Rest between bathing, dressing, and walking.
- Break activities into parts that can be done for a short time.
- Decide which activities are the most important to do. Decide which activities bring the most enjoyment or are necessary. Start with the most necessary or enjoyable activities.
- Get up or move slowly to avoid dizziness.
- Plan regular exercise to reduce fatigue.

- Eat a balanced diet with adequate protein. Eat from the four food groups (dairy products; fruits and vegetables; breads, cereals, rice, and pasta; proteins such as meat, chicken, fish, or eggs). The most important food group is carbohydrates, which provides energy most quickly. Examples of carbohydrates are pasta, potatoes, bread, fruit, and energy bars.
- Keep as active as possible during the day so that normal fatigue sets in at night.
- Resume patterns of rest and sleep as much as possible. Set regular times to nap and sleep so the body becomes used to a routine.
- Rest when tired by going to bed earlier, sleeping later, and taking naps during the day.
- Play relaxing music before sleep.
- Use some type of relaxation exercise before bedtime (see Chapter 7).
- Drink warm milk at bedtime.
- Take a warm bath or have a back rub at bedtime.
- Ask your doctor if you can take sleeping pills. (These medicines can cause problems when combined with other medications.)
- Do not force yourself to do more than you can manage.

CHAPTER 7

Complementary Nondrug Treatments

While going through cancer treatment, Daniel was bombarded with suggestions from friends about other methods he should try. Although people were just trying to help, it was confusing. He had also read a lot about complementary treatments, from relaxation and visualization to exercise and massage. He discussed all of these options with his doctor who was able to help him decide what might work best for him.

People may consider adding nonpharmacologic (nondrug) or complementary treatments for pain relief to use in conjunction with medications, surgery, or other medical procedures used for pain control. These therapies can be very useful in helping to reduce pain and manage side effects. They can be effectively used as part of a comprehensive pain management effort.

Complementary therapies can also help a person cope with the emotional and psychological impact of pain on an individual's quality of life and well being, both of which can be severely impacted by pain. For example, dealing with chronic pain can sometimes lead to depression or anxiety, which can make existing pain feel worse and decrease a person's desire to participate in family or social activities. It is clear that the mind can have a strong influence on the way a person deals with pain, whether positively or negatively. Because of this potentially powerful mind and body connection, it is important for physicians and patients to deal with the mind as well as the body and to consider the use of complementary techniques as part of a comprehensive effort to control pain.

The American Cancer Society (ACS) defines complementary treatments as supportive methods that are used to complement, or add to, conventional treatments. Complementary methods, such as massage therapy, yoga, and meditation are also referred to as nondrug or noninvasive treatments. These techniques rely heavily on the ability of the mind to influence responses to pain.

Complementary methods should not be confused with alternative therapies, which are unproven treatments sometimes used *instead of* conventional therapy to attempt to prevent, lessen, or cure disease. Alternative therapies may be harmful in and of themselves or because they are used instead of conventional medicine and thereby delay treatments that are proven to be helpful. *Complementary methods do not alter the growth or spread of cancer.*

Medicines for cancer pain are used to treat the sensation and perception of pain, that is, what you feel. Nondrug treatments are aimed at reducing the emotional

Questions to Ask About Complementary Nondrug Treatments

The following are some sample questions you may want to ask your doctor, other health professional, or licensed practitioner about any methods you are interested in pursuing for your pain.

Doctor or Health Care Professional:
- Are there any nondrug methods you recommend as a part of my cancer treatment in order to help me deal with pain or anxiety?
- What can I expect from this method or treatment?
- Is there any complementary method I should avoid?
- What kind of experience do you have with nondrug treatments?
- Does my hospital or medical facility offer this method? If not, where can I go to find out more about it?

components of pain as well as how people respond to pain. The benefits of many of these treatments are that they can increase a person's sense of personal control, reduce feelings of helplessness, provide opportunities to become actively involved in care, reduce stress and anxiety, elevate mood, and raise the pain threshold.

Techniques such as meditation or distraction are designed to target how the mind processes pain. These methods can help you learn how to relax and focus your thoughts away from the pain you are feeling, which lessens the effects of pain on your body. Skin stimulation, which includes the use of cold and heat, massage, and other elements, can be used to block pain sensations or alter blood flow in the parts of the body being stimulated. Complementary techniques, such as prayer and yoga, may also help reduce feelings of anxiety or depression, which can increase the intensity of cancer pain.

The psychological and physical benefits that can be gained from complementary nondrug treatments can have a very positive effect on your quality of life and well being. Many of these methods are also used during cancer treatment to help ease painful side effects or uncomfortable physical symptoms.

- Is the technique covered by my insurance? If not, what are the costs?
- Is this method widely available for use within the health care community, or is it controlled, with limited access to its use?

Licensed Practitioner:
- Are you licensed or trained in this method?
- How many years have you been practicing this method?
- Is this method difficult to master?
- Can I be taught this technique so that I can practice it at home on my own?
- Are there any risks involved?
- Are there any books, videos, or other resources available that you can recommend?

Access to Complementary Nondrug Treatments

Interest in therapies that tap into the connection between the mind and body, and its effects on healing and pain reduction, has grown in the medical community in recent years. Although research is still being done in this area, some treatments have been shown to be useful for dealing with cancer pain in particular as outlined in this chapter.

Many treatment centers recognize that therapies such as biofeedback, music therapy, and counseling can help people with cancer deal with pain and its impact on their quality of life. Some centers have begun to offer these therapies as part of a comprehensive cancer treatment program. Many complementary methods are also taught or administered by health professionals such as occupational and physical therapists, psychologists, social workers, or by other licensed and trained practitioners such as massage therapists, acupuncturists, clergy, or music therapists.

Some mind and body techniques, such as yoga and relaxation, can be self-taught and information is available through books, videos, and web sites. You may also find a class on some of these methods at fitness and community centers in your area, and some organizations can provide you with lists of licensed practitioners. The Resources section in the back of this book also contains contact information for some organizations.

When using complementary techniques, they should be incorporated as part of a comprehensive medical treatment plan that strives to help you deal with your cancer pain both mentally and physically. These methods can be safely used along with conventional treatment to help relieve symptoms or side effects, to ease pain, and to experience a better quality of life. Talk to members of your health care team about any nondrug treatments you are considering.

Complementary Nondrug Methods

The following techniques include methods that focus on the connections between the mind, body, and spirit, and their power for healing, as well as methods that involve touching, manipulation, or movement of the body. When used along with conventional treatment, many of these methods can help relieve pain or improve your quality of life.

ACUPUNCTURE

According to a National Institutes of Health (NIH) expert panel consisting of scientists, researchers, and health care providers, acupuncture is an effective treatment for nausea caused by chemotherapy drugs and for post-operative pain. Some evidence suggests that acupuncture may lessen the need for conventional pain relieving medicines.

Acupuncture is a technique in which very thin needles of varying lengths are inserted through the skin. In traditional acupuncture, specially trained practitioners insert needles at specific locations, called acupoints, which are believed to control specific areas of pain sensation. Needles usually remain in place for less than thirty minutes. Skilled acupuncturists cause virtually no pain. Once inserted, the acupuncturist may twirl the needles and apply heat or a weak electrical current to enhance the effects of therapy. In acupressure, a popular variation of acupuncture, therapists press on acupoints with their fingers instead of using needles. This technique is used by itself or as part of a larger system of manual healing such as in shiatsu massage.

Although it originated 2,000 to 3,000 years ago, acupuncture remains an important component of current traditional Chinese medicine. In China, acupuncture is used as an anesthetic during surgery and is believed to have the power to cure diseases and relieve symptoms of illness. Some practitioners claim that acupuncture relieves pain by stimulating the production of endorphins—natural substances in the body responsible for relieving pain. In the United States and Europe, it is used primarily to control pain and relieve disease symptoms such as nausea.

Many other conditions have been treated by acupuncture. The World Health Organization, for example, has listed more than forty diseases that lend themselves to acupuncture treatment. They noted that the list is based on clinical experience rather than research findings.[1] The NIH states that acupuncture may be useful as an adjunct treatment (used in addition to the main treatment) for conditions such as addiction, stroke rehabilitation, headache, menstrual cramps, tennis elbow, fibromyalgia, myofacial pain, osteoarthritis, low back pain, carpal tunnel syndrome, and asthma. However, further research is needed to determine the effectiveness for its use with these and other conditions.

[1] World Health Organization 1979, World Health Magazine, p. 27.

Acupuncture is considered useful when treating conditions for which it has been proven to be effective (e.g., nausea and vomiting caused by chemotherapy, and postoperative pain). However, the NIH has not specifically recommended using acupuncture for cancer pain.

Most doctors believe acupuncture is safe as long as the needles used are sterile and the therapy is conducted by a trained professional. The American Academy of Medical Acupuncture maintains a current referral list of doctors who practice acupuncture. Medicare does not cover acupuncture, but it is covered by some private health insurance plans and health maintenance organizations.

BIOFEEDBACK

Biofeedback is a treatment method that uses monitoring devices to help people consciously regulate physiological (bodily) processes that are usually controlled automatically, such as heart rate, blood pressure, temperature, perspiration, and muscle tension. It has been approved by an independent panel convened by the NIH as a useful complementary therapy for treating chronic pain and insomnia. Biofeedback can also be used to regulate or alter other physical functions that may be causing discomfort. Mastering these responses allows one to reduce pain and make other positive changes. For the person with chronic cancer-related pain, biofeedback might be used along with effective pain relieving medicines.

With the help of special monitoring devices that provide feedback, people can learn to control certain body functions such as heart rate, blood pressure, and muscle tension. A biofeedback therapist uses these monitoring devices to measure information that controls bodily processes. Messages are sent to the person that indicate when the desired results occur. The process is repeated as often as necessary until a person can reliably use conscious thought to change physical functions.

There are several different ways to measure body functions for biofeedback:

- Electromyogram (EMG) measures muscle tension. It is used to help heal muscle injuries and relieve chronic pain.
- Thermal biofeedback provides information about skin temperature, which is a good indicator of blood flow. Several health problems are related to blood flow, such as migraine headaches, anxiety, and high blood pressure.

- Electrodermal activity (EDA) shows changes in perspiration rates. It is used in treating anxiety.
- Finger pulse measurements are used to reflect high blood pressure, heart beat irregularities, and anxiety.
- Breathing rate is monitored to promote relaxation.

By learning to control heart rates, skin temperature, breathing rates, muscle control, and other physiological activity in the body, biofeedback can reduce stress and muscle tension from a variety of causes. Through a greater awareness of bodily functions, it can regulate or alter other physical functions that may cause discomfort.

Biofeedback may also be useful in retraining muscles after injury, or teaching new muscles to take over. Perhaps the greatest benefit of biofeedback you may experience is the ability to reduce tension and promote relaxation, both of which can help you cope with your cancer pain.

Biofeedback requires a trained and certified professional to control monitoring equipment and interpret changes. Check with your medical facility to see if they offer biofeedback therapy.

DISTRACTION

Distraction is a technique used to turn a person's attention to something other than the pain that he or she may be feeling. When used along with effective pain medicines, distraction can help decrease anxiety, pain, fatigue, and muscle tension. It can also increase confidence in the ability to handle pain. Because this technique does not require much energy, it may be useful when a person is tired. Slow, rhythmic breathing can also be used for distraction as well as for relaxation.

Many people use this method without realizing it when they watch television or listen to the radio to "take their minds off" the pain. When listening to music, the volume can be adjusted to match the intensity of pain, making it louder for very severe pain. Some people find it helpful to listen to fast music through a headset or earphones. To help keep your attention on the music you can tap out the rhythm.

Any activity that occupies your attention can be used for distraction. For example, losing yourself in a good book or going to a movie might divert your mind from pain. If your concentration is diminished, you may try math games, like subtracting 4 from 1,000, or counting back from a certain number. If you enjoy working with your hands, crafts such as needlework, model building, or painting may be useful in distracting you from pain.

After using a distraction technique, some people report that they are tired, irritable, and feel more pain. Some people think that a person who can be distracted from pain does not have severe pain. This is not necessarily true. If these are problems for you, you may want to use distraction carefully or privately. You can find out more about this technique by asking someone on your health care team or by contacting the ACS.

EXERCISE

Exercise is the performance of physical activity that requires energy expenditure. It is important for people to exercise regularly to keep muscles functioning as well as possible. Regular exercise can help increase your energy level, reduce pain, and contribute to your well being. Exercise can also prevent problems associated with immobility, such as stiff joints, breathing problems, constipation, skin sores, poor appetite, and mental changes.

Aerobic exercise (such as walking, jogging, cycling, yoga, and swimming) increases blood flow to the heart and oxygen to the lungs. Regular aerobic exercise can also lower blood cholesterol, strengthen bones, raise metabolism, and increase endurance. *Anaerobic* exercise (such as strength training) is essential for developing muscles, strength, speed, and power, and for maintaining freedom of movement. An ideal exercise program should combine aerobic and anaerobic exercises.

The ACS recommends thirty minutes of regular exercise several times a week. The thirty minutes does not need to be continuous to be beneficial. You can accomplish this goal of thirty minutes by walking briskly (three to four miles per hour) for about two miles or by a variety of other activities, including jogging, swimming, gardening, housework, or dancing at a level of intensity equivalent to brisk walking. It's important when exercising to try to maintain a positive attitude, set reasonable goals, and stick to a regular exercise program.

Some form of physical activity is beneficial to everyone, even someone confined to a bed. Range of motion exercises and general stretching can be performed quite easily. In fact, pain medication combined with stretching exercises is one of the best solutions for keeping comfortable when confined to bed.

Inactivity can lead to muscle weakness, pain in joints or legs, and other problems such as poor or no appetite, constipation, skin sores, problems with breathing, and mental changes. Performing range-of-motion exercises as instructed by your nurse, doctor, or physical therapist can help alleviate some of these problems.

Exercise can provide benefits to your mind as well as your body. Physical activities may improve your sense of being in touch with your body. Regular exercise can also induce feelings of relaxation and optimism and may help decrease feelings of inadequacy and helplessness. For many people, exercise provides a sense of accomplishment and control—this is especially helpful to people who may be feeling depressed. Exercise also has a calming affect on many people and can be a form of distraction from pain.

Before you begin an exercise program, talk with your doctor who will take into account your particular circumstances so that a program of exercise can be tailored to your situation. This will allow you to learn the types of exercise best for maintaining your health, the level of activity appropriate for you, and signs to watch for that might indicate overexertion. Pushing yourself too hard may be discouraging and could result in injury. Be aware that some treatments limit physical activity. Be sure to ask about activities you should avoid. Your doctor should be able to recommend an exercise professional or physical therapist to help you get started. You can also check with the YWCA (212-273-7800), YMCA (888-333-YMCA), or American Heart Association (800-AHA-USA1) for information on exercise programs.

HUMOR THERAPY

The dictionary defines humor as comical or amusing entertainment, or a quality that appeals to the sense of the ridiculous. Humor therapy is the use of humor for the relief of physical and emotional difficulties. It is used as a technique to promote health and cope with illness. Laughter can stimulate the circulatory system by increasing heart rate and oxygen use.

Humor has been used in medicine throughout recorded history. One of the earliest mentions of the health benefits of humor is in the book of Proverbs in the Bible. As early as the 13th century, some surgeons used humor to distract patients from the pain of surgery. Humor was also widely used and studied by the medical community in the early 20th century. In more modern times, the most famous story of humor therapy involved Norman Cousins, then editor of the *Saturday Review*. According to the story, Mr. Cousins "cured" himself from an unknown illness with a self-invented regimen of laughter and vitamins.

For many people, humor therapy can provide a welcome distraction from pain. It is useful for treating people with physical and emotional problems. It is generally used to improve quality of life, provide some pain relief, encourage relaxation, and reduce stress. It is thought that being able to find humor in everyday events can be helpful. As with so many mind and body connections, humor seems to provide temporary relief from worry and can lead to an overall sense of well being. Physically, laughter exercises the same muscles and organs we use for breathing, promoting relaxation and reducing stress. The use of humor can sometimes lead to an increase in pain tolerance.

Many hospitals and ambulatory care centers have incorporated special rooms where materials—and sometimes people—are used to help make people laugh. Materials include movies, audio and videotapes, books, games, and puzzles for patients of every age. Many hospitals also use volunteer groups who visit patients for the purpose of providing opportunities for laughter.

HYPNOSIS

Hypnosis is one of several relaxation methods that has been approved by an independent panel, convened by the NIH, as a useful complementary therapy for treating chronic pain. People with cancer can use hypnosis to reduce pain, promote relaxation, and reduce stress. Hypnosis can also lower blood pressure and anxiety, and be used to reduce nausea, vomiting, phobias, and aversions to certain cancer treatments. People who are hypnotized have selective attention, and are able to achieve a state of heightened concentration while blocking out distractions. Under hypnosis, people can achieve a state of restful alertness that helps them focus on a certain problem or symptom. This allows them to be open to images, suggestions, and ideas for resolving issues and improving their quality of life.

There are many different types of hypnotic techniques, however, most hypnosis begins with an induction. While a person is sitting or lying quietly, the hypnotherapist talks in gentle, soothing tones, describes images, and repeats a series of verbal suggestions that allow a person to become relaxed, yet deeply absorbed and focused on their awareness. People under hypnosis may appear to be asleep, but they are actually in an altered state of concentration and can focus on a specific goal. During hypnosis, a person is very receptive to suggestions made by the hypnotherapist. To relieve pain, the therapist may suggest that pain will be gone when the person "wakes up." Some cancer patients have learned methods of self-hypnosis that they use to control pain.

Contrary to what many believe, people under hypnosis are not under the control of the hypnotherapist nor can they be made to do something they do not want to do. Hypnosis will not work if the person does not want to be hypnotized. Hypnosis is not brainwashing and ideas are not "planted" in people's minds to make people do things against their will. Quite the opposite is true. Hypnosis is used to help people gain more control over their actions, emotions, and bodies. The ability to block a natural response through intense concentration makes hypnosis a good pain reliever for painful medical experiences.

Health care professionals including physicians, psychotherapists, and social workers can perform hypnosis. People who practice hypnosis are licensed. It is important to be hypnotized by a trained professional. Ask your doctor for more information about where to find a qualified hypnotherapist or contact the American Society for Clinical Hypnosis (312-645-9810).

IMAGERY AND VISUALIZATION

Imagery involves the use of mental exercises and relaxation techniques designed to enable the mind to influence the health and well being of the body. It is like a deliberate daydream that actively involves all of the senses. Imagery is considered to be similar to meditation (see page 155). Some people have found that imagery can relieve physical pain and emotional anxiety, improve the effectiveness of drug therapies, and provide emotional insights. Imagery is also used in biofeedback and hypnosis.

Some people with cancer use imagery to reduce the nausea and vomiting associated with chemotherapy, to relieve stress, enhance the immune system, promote weight gain, and fight depression. It is also thought that certain images may reduce pain both during imagery and for hours afterward, although it is not completely understood how it works.

There are a variety of imagery techniques. One common technique, guided imagery, involves visualizing a specific image or goal to be achieved and then imagining achieving that goal. Guided imagery can be helpful in managing stress, anxiety, and depression, and in lowering blood pressure, pain, and the side effects

Imagery Exercise for Pain

Ball of Energy

The following is an exercise using the image of a ball of energy. It is a variation of the technique credited to Dr. David Bresler at the Pain Control Unit, University of California, Los Angeles (UCLA).

- Close your eyes. Breathe slowly and feel yourself relax.
- Concentrate on your breathing. Breathe slowly and comfortably from your abdomen. Breathe in this slow rhythm for a few minutes.
- Imagine a ball of healing energy forming in your lungs or on your chest. It may be like a white light. It can be vague. It does not have to be vivid. Imagine this ball forming, taking shape. Sometimes imaging pouring cool water on a burning pain or sensation is useful.
- When you are ready, imagine that the air you breathe in blows this healing ball of energy to the area of your pain. Once there, the ball heals and relaxes you.
- When you breathe out, imagine the air blows the ball away from your body. As it goes, the ball takes your pain with it. (Be careful: do not blow as you breathe out. Breathe out naturally.)
- Repeat the last two steps each time you breathe in and out.
- You may imagine that the ball gets bigger and bigger as it takes more and more discomfort away from your body.
- To end the imagery, count slowly to three, breathe in deeply, open your eyes, and say silently to yourself, "I feel alert and relaxed."
- Begin moving about slowly.

of chemotherapy. It can also be valuable in easing anxiety related to radiation therapy, including fears about the equipment, surgical pain, and recurrence of cancer. Imagery for pain relief is usually done with the eyes closed. A relaxation technique may be used first. The image can be something such as a ball of healing energy or a picture drawn in your mind of yourself as a person without pain.

Imagery techniques can be learned with the help of books and tapes, or they can be practiced under the guidance of a trained therapist. Imagery sessions with a health professional may last twenty to thirty minutes. Ask your nurse or doctor if information about imagery techniques is available at your medical facility.

MEDITATION

Meditation is a mind-body method that uses concentration or reflection to relax the body and calm the mind in order to create a sense of well being. To meditate is to ponder, to think about, or to reflect upon. The ultimate goal of meditation is to separate oneself mentally from the outside world. The NIH National Center for Complementary and Alternative Medicine reports that regular meditation can increase longevity and the quality of life; and reduce chronic pain, anxiety, high blood pressure, substance abuse, and blood cortisol levels initially brought on by stress.

Meditation can be a helpful relaxation method when used as a complementary method for treating chronic pain and some of the side effects of pain including insomnia, stress, and anxiety. Successful meditation can result in clearing the mind of all distractions, including those that create stress, discomfort, worry, and fear, all of which can increase the sensation of pain for people with cancer.

According to practitioners, meditation should be performed once or twice a day for fifteen to twenty minutes. A quiet room where a person can sit comfortably is needed. Typically, a meditator will sit with closed eyes and attempt to achieve a feeling of peace until a relaxed yet alert state is reached. To reach this state, a person will concentrate on a pleasant idea or thought, chant a phrase or special sound (sometimes called a mantra), or focus on the sound of his or her own breathing. Although meditation is usually done while sitting, there are some forms which involve movement like tai chi, aikido (a Japanese martial art), and walking (in Zen Buddhism).

Meditation can be performed without an instructor or it can be guided by yoga masters, doctors, or mental health professionals such as psychiatrists. Some clinics at major medical centers and local hospitals practice meditation as a form of behavioral medicine. Information about meditation can also be found in books and videotapes.

MUSIC THERAPY

Music therapy is a method that consists of the active or passive use of music in order to promote healing and enhance the quality of life. There is some evidence that when used along with conventional medical treatment, music therapy can help to reduce pain and anxiety, and relieve chemotherapy-induced nausea and vomiting. It may also relieve stress and provide an overall sense of well being, which can be important factors for a person living with chronic pain. Some medical experts believe music can aid healing and improve physical movement. Music therapy may also reduce high blood pressure, rapid heartbeat, breathing rate, depression, and sleeplessness.

Some aspects of music therapy include music improvisation, receptive music listening, songwriting, lyric discussion, imagery, music performance, and learning through music. Individuals can also perform their own music therapy by listening to music or sounds at home.

Music therapists design sessions for individuals and groups based on individual needs and tastes. Music therapy can be conducted in a variety of places, including hospitals, cancer centers, hospices, at home, or anywhere people can benefit from its calming or stimulating effects.

There are currently over 5,000 professional music therapists working in health care settings in the United States today. They serve as part of cancer-management teams in many hospitals and cancer centers, helping to plan and evaluate treatment. Check with the American Music Therapy Association for more information (www.namt.com).

PSYCHOTHERAPY/COUNSELING

Psychotherapy, also referred to as counseling, covers a wide range of approaches designed to help people change their ways of thinking, feeling, or behaving. It may improve a person's quality of life by helping to reduce anxiety and depression, both of which can accompany pain and affect a person's sense of well being. Therapy can also be beneficial for family members of people with cancer to help them deal with such feelings as anxiety or helplessness.

Psychotherapy can help you develop more effective coping strategies for dealing with cancer and some of its side effects such as pain and stress. It can also teach you ways to communicate better with your doctor and allow you to more closely follow medical instructions because you feel your own needs are being recognized. Therapy may be conducted individually, as well as in couples, families, and groups (see Chapter 8).

RELAXATION

Relaxation exercises are used to relieve some types of pain, or to keep it from getting worse by reducing tension in the muscles. They can increase energy, reduce fatigue and anxiety, promote sleep, and make other pain relief methods work better. For example, some people find that relaxation techniques enhance the effectiveness of pain medication or cold/hot packs.

There are a number of different relaxation methods. *Visual concentration* involves opening your eyes and staring at an object, or closing your eyes and thinking of a peaceful, calm scene. *Rhythmic massage* is done with the palm of your hand by massaging an area of pain in a circular, firm manner. *Inhaling* and *exhaling* involve breathing in deeply while tensing your muscles or a group of muscles, then holding your breath and keeping muscles tense for a second or two, and then letting go and breathing out while letting your body go limp. You can practice *slow rhythmic breathing* by staring at an object, or by closing your eyes and concentrating on your breathing or on a peaceful scene. Other methods include using *imagery* (see Imagery in this chapter), listening to slow, familiar music through an earphone or headset, and *progressive muscle relaxation* which involves learning how to relax different muscle groups throughout your body.

Relaxation may be practiced sitting up or lying down. Choose a quiet place whenever possible. Close your eyes. Do not cross your arms and legs because that may cut off circulation and cause numbness or tingling. If you are lying down, be sure you are comfortable; it will not work if it is forced. It may take up to two weeks of practice to feel the first results of relaxation. It should be practiced for at least five to ten minutes twice a day.

Relaxation may be difficult to use with severe pain. However, you may be able to use a simple relaxation method such as visual concentration with rhythmic massage or breathe in/tense, breathe out/relax. Sometimes breathing too deeply for a while can cause shortness of breath. If this is a problem, take shallow breaths and/or breathe more slowly. If you experience a feeling of "suffocation," take a deep breath and exhale slowly, trying not to focus on your breathing. *Do not continue any relaxation technique that increases your pain, makes you feel uneasy, or causes any unpleasant effects.*

Relaxation Exercises You Can Try

Visual concentration and rhythmic massage:

- Open your eyes and stare at an object, or close your eyes and think of a peaceful, calm scene.
- With the palm of your hand, massage near the area of pain in a circular, firm manner. Avoid red, raw, swollen, or tender areas. You may wish to ask a family member or friend to do this for you.

Inhale/tense, exhale/relax:

- Inhale (breathe in) deeply. At the same time, tense your muscles or a group of muscles. For example, you can squeeze your eyes shut, frown, clench your teeth, make a fist, or stiffen your arms and legs as tightly as you can.
- Hold your breath and keep muscles tense for a second or two.
- Let go! Exhale (breathe out) and let your body go limp.

Slow rhythmic breathing:

- Stare at an object or close your eyes and concentrate on your breathing or on a peaceful scene.
- Take a slow, deep breath.
- As you breathe out, relax your muscles and feel the tension draining.
- Now remain relaxed and begin breathing slowly and comfortably, concentrating on your breathing. Just breathe naturally. If you ever feel out of breath, take a deep breath and then continue the slow breathing exercise. Each time you breathe out, feel yourself relaxing and going limp. If some muscles are not relaxed such as your shoulders, focus on them and relax them as you breathe out. You need to do this only once or twice for each specific muscle group.
- Continue slow, rhythmic breathing for a few seconds up to ten minutes, depending on your need.
- To end your slow rhythmic breathing, count silently and slowly from one to three. Open your eyes. Say silently to yourself, "I feel alert and relaxed." Begin moving about slowly.

There are various relaxation tapes commercially available that can provide step-by-step instructions in relaxation techniques. If you have trouble using these methods, ask your doctor or nurse to refer you to a therapist who is experienced in relaxation techniques.

SKIN STIMULATION
(Cold and Heat, Massage, Menthol, Pressure, and Vibration)

Skin stimulation is the use of pressure, friction, temperature change, or chemical substances to excite the nerve endings in the skin. Scientists believe that the same nerve pathways transmit the sensations of pain directly to the brain. When the skin is stimulated so that pressure, warmth, or cold is felt, pain sensation is lessened or blocked. Skin stimulation also alters the flow of blood to the affected area. Sometimes skin stimulation will get rid of the pain, or the pain will be lessened during the stimulation and for hours after it is finished.

Stimulation is done either on or near the area of pain. You also can use skin stimulation on the side of the body opposite of the pain. For example, you might stimulate the left knee to decrease pain in the right knee. Stimulating the skin in areas away from the pain can be used to increase relaxation and may relieve pain.

Cold or Heat Applications

Cold applications are often used to reduce pain by numbing the affected area with gel packs or ice. Gel packs work well because they are soft and flexible (even at freezing temperatures) and can be reused as often as necessary. An ice pack or ice cubes wrapped in a towel can also be effective. Gel packs are available at drugstores and medical supply stores.

Heat applications are generally used to soothe painful or sore muscles. A heating pad that generates its own moisture (hydrocolater) is useful for this purpose. Other heat applications include heated gel packs, hot water bottles, hot towels, a regular heating pad, or a hot bath or shower.

It is important to remember that heat and cold applications can easily damage skin. Extreme heat or cold can burn your skin. When using either method, you should limit your exposure to five to ten minutes and do not use any application over any area where your circulation or sensation is poor.

Massage

A growing number of health care professionals recognize massage as a useful addition to conventional medical treatment. Massage can relieve stress, anxiety, and pain. It involves manipulating, rubbing, and kneading the body's muscle and soft tissue. For pain relief, it is most effective when slow, steady, circular motions are used. Massage can be applied over or near the area of pain with bare hands or with any substance that feels good such as talcum powder, warm oil, or hand lotion. Depending upon where your pain is located, you may do it yourself or ask a family member or friend to give you a massage. Having someone give you a foot rub, back rub, or hand rub can be very relaxing and may relieve pain. Some people find brushing or stroking lightly more comforting than deep massage. Use whatever works best for you.

There is a wide range of training and certification available for massage therapists. Not all states require licensing, but it may be helpful to use a massage therapist who has experience and training in helping clients who suffer from cancer pain.

Menthol

Many menthol preparations are available for pain relief. When they are rubbed into the skin, they increase blood circulation to the affected area and produce a warm (sometimes cool) soothing feeling that lasts for several hours. There are creams, lotions, liniments, or gels that contain menthol. Brands include Ben-Gay, Icy Hot, Mineral Ice, and Heat.

Before using a menthol preparation over a large area, test a small amount of the preparation in a circle about one inch in diameter in the area of pain (or the area to be stimulated). This will let you know whether the menthol is uncomfortable to you or irritates your skin.

Pressure

Pressure can be applied with the entire hand or the base, the fingertip, knuckle, or the ball of the thumb. It is usually most effective when applied as firmly as possible without causing pain. You can use pressure for up to one minute. This often will relieve pain for several minutes to several hours after the pressure is released.

You may want to experiment by applying pressure for about ten seconds to various areas over or near your pain to see if it helps. You can also feel around

Some Warnings About
the Use of Skin Stimulation

- If skin stimulation increases your pain, stop using it.
- Avoid massage and vibration over red, raw, tender, or swollen areas.
- If you are having radiation therapy, check with your doctor or nurse before using skin stimulation. You should not apply ointments, salves, or liniments to the treatment area, and you should not use heat or extreme cold on treated areas. You should also avoid massage in the treated area.
- Many menthol preparations contain an ingredient similar to aspirin. A small amount of this aspirin-like substance is absorbed through the skin. If you have been told not to take aspirin, do not use these preparations until you check with your doctor.
- Do not rub menthol preparations over broken skin, a skin rash, or mucous membranes (such as inside your mouth or around your rectum). Make sure you do not get the menthol in your eyes.
- Do not use heat over a new injury because it can increase bleeding. Wait at least twenty-four hours.
- Never use a heating pad on bare skin or go to sleep with it turned on. Be careful while using a heating pad if you do not have much feeling in the area on which you are using it.
- Do not use cold so intense or for so long that the cold itself causes pain. If you start to shiver when using cold, stop using it right away.

your pain and outward to see if you can find "trigger points," small areas under the skin that are especially sensitive or that trigger pain.

Vibration

Vibration can also be used to bring temporary relief over or near an area of pain. For example, the scalp attachment of a hand-held vibrator often relieves a headache. For low back pain, a vibrator placed at the small of the back may be helpful. You may also use a vibrating device such as a small battery-operated vibrator, a hand-held electric vibrator, a large heat-massage electric pad, a bed vibrator, or a vibrating chair. These devices can usually be found at your local drug store or medical supply store.

Some of the stimulation methods listed above may be helpful in reducing your pain. You may want to experiment with different methods to see which ones work best for you. If you are not sure which you should or should not try, talk to your nurse or doctor about your options.

SPIRITUALITY AND PRAYER

Spirituality is generally described as an awareness of something greater than the individual and is usually expressed through religion or prayer. Spirituality and religion are very important to the quality of life for some people with cancer. Intercessory prayer (praying for others) may be an effective addition to conventional medical care. The benefits of prayer may include reduction of stress and anxiety, promotion of a more positive outlook, and the strengthening of the will to live, all of which can have a significant impact on the life of a person dealing with chronic pain.

People who practice various forms of spirituality claim that prayer can decrease the negative effects of disease (such as pain), speed recovery, and increase the effectiveness of medical treatments. Because the pain and side effects of cancer may be overwhelming, regular participation in spiritual practices such as prayer can help to provide better coping skills and enhance well being for some people. Religious attendance has been associated with improvement of various health conditions such as cancer, as well as overall health status.

There are many forms of spirituality. The most common involve prayer and regular attendance at religious ceremonies (usually at churches, synagogues, or temples). Prayer, which can be performed alone or in a group, may be silent or spoken out loud and can take place in any setting. Spirituality in the form of religious attendance may also involve praying for one's self or for others. In this type of setting, the entire congregation of a church may be asked to pray for a sick person or the person's family. Some religions set aside certain times of the day and special days of the week for prayer. Standard prayers written by religious leaders are often memorized and repeated during private sessions and in groups. Prayers often ask a higher being for help, understanding, wisdom, or strength in dealing with life's problems.

Many medical institutions and practitioners include spirituality and prayer as important components of healing. In addition, hospitals have chapels, and they contract with ministers, rabbis, and voluntary organizations to serve the spiritual needs of people with cancer. Information about local churches or other religious organizations in your area should be available in your local phone directory.

TRANSCUTANEOUS ELECTRICAL NERVE STIMULATION (TENS)

Transcutaneous electrical nerve stimulation (TENS) is a method of pain relief in which a special device transmits electrical impulses through electrodes to an area of the body that is in pain. Drs. Ronald Melzac and Patrick Wall developed the Gate Control Theory of Pain in 1965, which claims that when nerves are electrically stimulated, a gate mechanism is closed in the spinal cord preventing the awareness of pain. After the introduction of the theory, TENS was widely used to treat pain.

Supporters claim that TENS is an effective method for relieving acute pain caused by surgery, migraines, injuries, arthritis, tendonitis, bursitis, chronic wounds, cancer, and other sources. Some cancer patients, particularly those with mild neuropathic pain (pain related to nerve tissue damage), may benefit from TENS for brief periods of time. TENS may also be more effective when used with analgesics (pain medicines). Although there is some evidence that TENS may offer short-term pain relief for some people, the long-term benefits have not been proven.

A TENS system consists of an electrical generator connected by wires to a pair of electrodes. The electrodes are attached to the patient's skin near the source of pain. When the generator is switched on, a mild electrical current travels through the electrodes into the body. Patients may feel tingling or warmth during treatment. A session typically lasts from five to fifteen minutes and treatments may be applied as often as necessary, depending on the severity of pain.

TENS is used widely by physical therapists and other medical practitioners, but can also be performed at home by patients using a portable TENS system. There are more than one hundred types of TENS units approved for use by the Food and Drug Administration. A prescription is needed to obtain a system, so if you are interested in obtaining a home TENS unit, you will need to talk to your doctor or physical therapist.

YOGA

Yoga is a form of nonaerobic exercise that involves a program of precise posture and breathing activities. Yoga is one of the oldest mind and body health systems in existence and was first practiced in India over 5,000 years ago. According to a report to the NIH, there is some evidence to suggest yoga may be useful as a complementary method to help relieve symptoms associated with cancer, asthma, diabetes, drug addiction, high blood pressure, heart disease, and migraine headaches. Research has also shown that yoga can be used to control physiological functions such as heart rate, respiration, metabolism, body temperature, brain waves, skin resistance, and other bodily functions.

People who practice yoga claim that it leads to a state of physical health, relaxation, happiness, peace, and tranquility. There is some evidence showing that yoga can lower stress, increase strength, and provide a good form of exercise. Proponents also claim that yoga can be used to eliminate insomnia and increase stamina. Yoga may help a person with cancer pain to enjoy an enhanced quality of life through better physical fitness and increased relaxation techniques.

Tips About Complementary Nondrug Treatments

- In order to avoid injury or increased pain, consult your doctor before beginning any exercise that may involve the manipulation of joints and muscles.
- Ask your doctor if he or she can recommend a certain complementary therapy that can help you with your particular kind of pain.
- Some insurance and health plans will cover at least some of the costs of several complementary techniques, such as acupuncture, biofeedback, and hypnosis because these methods can be helpful in reducing pain and other side effects of treatment.
- Contact the National Institutes of Health National Center for Complementary and Alternative Medicine for more information (888-644-6226).

There are different variations and aspects of yoga. The most common form of yoga involves the use of movement, breathing exercises, and meditation to achieve a connection with the mind, body, and spirit. The goal of yoga is perfect concentration to attain the ancient Hindu ideal of samadhi—separation of pure consciousness from the outside world through the development of intuitive insight.

Practitioners claim yoga should be done either at the beginning or end of the day. A yoga session starts with the person sitting in an upright position and performing gentle movements, all of which are executed very slowly, while taking slow, deep breaths from the abdomen. Yoga can be practiced at home without an instructor, or in adult education classes, health clubs, and community centers. There are also numerous books and videotapes available. A typical session can last between twenty minutes to one hour. A yoga session may include guided relaxation, meditation, and sometimes visualization. It often ends with the chanting of a mantra (a meaningful word or phrase) to achieve a deeper state of relaxation. Yoga requires several sessions a week in order to become proficient.

Some yoga postures are difficult to achieve. *Consult your doctor before beginning any exercise that may involve the manipulation of joints and muscles.*

CHAPTER 8

Coping with the Emotional and Social Impact of Cancer Pain

"There is a fear that goes through you when you are told you have cancer. It's so hard in the beginning to think about anything but your diagnosis. It's the first thing you think about every morning. I want people diagnosed with cancer to know it does get better. Talking about your cancer helps you deal with all of the new emotions you are feeling. Remember it's normal to get upset."

Delores, a cancer survivor

Quality of Life

Pain is not a purely physical experience. It can profoundly affect all aspects of emotional health. Pain can also interfere with your normal daily activities. Pain diminishes the enjoyment of everyday pleasures, prevents relaxation and sleep, and increases anxiety, stress, and fatigue. It may cause feelings of helplessness, depression, isolation, anger, and worry, and often makes people withdraw. Individuals who experience continuous mild or moderate pain often report that their social activities decrease and that they have less contact with friends and family. In other words, pain affects your quality of life.

Pain may even cause guilt when patients believe they are being punished for something they've done or when they think they depend too much on friends or family. As the intensity and duration of pain increase, so does its negative impact on a good quality of life. Severe and unrelenting pain can become all-consuming and can completely immobilize an individual. Constant pain intrudes on every aspect of a person's life.

When the source of pain is cancer, the psychological impact is magnified by the sudden reality of facing a serious illness and confronting a life crisis. Physical pain can intensify emotions evoked by a diagnosis of cancer, such as fear, anxiety, worry, and depression. In one research study,[1] cancer patients who attributed new pain to a source other than cancer reported less interference in daily activities and pleasure than those who believed the new pain came from progression of their disease. Another study[2] found that women with metastatic breast cancer experienced more discomfort when they believed new pain was a sign their cancer had spread and if they were depressed. In comparison, less anxious and depressed people with cancer reported less pain. In a third research study,[3] patients who reported negative thoughts about their personal or social skills reported more pain and emotional distress than those who viewed themselves as more socially independent. Clearly, much research demonstrates that the physical and psychological factors of pain and cancer are linked.

Pain is one of the most important factors that affects the quality of life among people with cancer. For this reason, reducing or eliminating cancer-related pain is important. Pain relief often results in fewer emotional and psychological problems, improved outlook and mood, greater optimism about the future, and greater ability to cope with cancer and cancer treatment.

MEASURING QUALITY OF LIFE

Some of the factors that make up quality of life can be easily measured, such as strength and functional abilities, like walking, sleeping, and eating independently. Other factors, such as depression, anxiety, and the quality of relationships with friends and loved ones, can also be measured.

Only the person with cancer knows the amount or type of pain experienced and how it affects daily life. The patient is the best judge of how pain feels.

[1] R. L. Daut, and C. S. Cleeland, "The Prevalence and Severity of Pain in Cancer," *Cancer*, 50 (1982): 1913-1918.
[2] D. Spiegel, and J. R. Bloom, "Pain in Metastatic Breast Cancer," *Cancer*, 52 (1983): 341-345.
[3] D. Payne, "Cognition in Cancer Pain," Ph.D. diss, University of Louisville, Louisville Ky., 1995.

Ingredients of the Quality of Life

Researchers have identified four key components that constitute quality of life:
- *Physical* well being includes things like strength, mobility, and fatigue.
- *Psychological* well being includes feelings like happiness, sadness, anxiety, and fear.
- *Interpersonal* well being includes relationships with family, friends, and caregivers.
- *Spiritual* well being includes the meaning of suffering and the purpose of life.

Caregivers need to rely on the person's description of pain. Research has shown that self-reporting is a more accurate gauge of pain than observations from medical personnel or caregivers at home. Doubting the person's report of pain creates anxiety and mistrust, which can worsen pain.

Common Feelings Related to Cancer and Cancer Pain

Most people initially feel tremendous emotional upheaval after being diagnosed with cancer. They may experience many painful feelings such as disbelief, shock, fear, and anger. It is often hard to absorb all of the information about the cancer in the midst of all those feelings. It takes time to accept and understand the diagnosis.

People cope with cancer in different ways. Through time, most survivors come to terms with the reality of living with a diagnosis of cancer. After the initial shock of diagnosis and the beginning of treatment, most people find that they are able to continue much of their normal lives. They learn to adapt and continue with work, entertainment, and social relationships. Many cancer survivors say that being diagnosed with cancer gave them an opportunity to re-evaluate their lives and find strengths and abilities they did not know they had. Of course there are times when finding strength is hard and the situation feels overwhelming.

Research shows that pain causes significant psychological distress. On the other hand, mental outlook has a big impact on how a person perceives and copes with pain. People with cancer who are depressed or anxious typically report more pain than those who are calm and optimistic. Those whose daily activities are impaired by cancer and its treatment and who rely on caregivers for help also report more pain than those who are self-sufficient.

Feelings and attitudes about pain may also be influenced by culture, age, and gender (see Chapter 1). In some cultures, complaining about pain is not encouraged, so patients suffer in silence even when pain relief is available. In other cultural groups, people in pain may be more vocal about their pain and insist on relief. Men are often raised to be "tough" and remain silent about pain. In general, women are more likely to acknowledge the presence of pain and ask for help. Similarly, older people are less likely than younger people to complain about pain.

For many people with cancer, pain signals that cancer has spread or is getting worse, though this is not necessarily true. This belief can lead to anxiety and depression, which must be considered by the health care team when planning pain control strategies. Learning how to cope with these symptoms can effectively reduce a person's level of pain.

INDIVIDUAL REACTIONS TO PAIN

Predicting how any one individual will cope with cancer pain is difficult. Everyone reacts differently. Some people may be able to carry on normal activities, even when in moderate pain. Others may be incapacitated by the same level of pain. This doesn't mean that one person is tougher than another, only that there is a wide variation in the way we react to and deal with pain.

Functional limitations such as difficulty walking, eating, or sleeping, or being unable to take care of oneself may affect one person's outlook on life far differently than it affects another. People whose pain keeps them from moving about comfortably may experience strong psychological reactions, such as hopelessness. Yet the same restrictions may cause minimal distress if they are comfortable relying on others for help. One person may benefit most from pain treatment that allows more mobility, while another may be satisfied with a pain level that permits better sleep.

The degree of an individual's psychological distress depends on many factors, such as social support, coping ability, and personality. Pain complicates the picture further. Pain relief usually helps people cope more effectively with stress and deal with the reality of cancer and the implications of the disease.

A person's spirituality, or beliefs in a higher power, may affect or be affected by pain. Some people find that religious observance or worship calms and soothes them, thereby decreasing perceptions of pain. For others, the social interaction offered by organized religious groups provides a strong support network and social outlet. Still others may feel abandoned and isolated if they believe that their faith has failed them.

PAIN AND DEPRESSION

Some degree of frustration and discouragement is common when people are coping with cancer-related pain. Clinical depression, a treatable condition, occurs in about 25 percent of people with cancer. It causes a person to feel hopeless, unmotivated, and less able to follow treatment demands. Depression can occur as a side effect of some medicines, or it can be caused by unrelieved pain. Depression can also develop as a response to the treatment and diagnosis of cancer.

Depression often affects sleep, appetite, and energy level. It may rob a person of the feeling of pleasure in life. It also tends to intensify the person's perception of pain. People with cancer who are clinically depressed report greater pain severity than nondepressed people. People in pain are also more likely to become depressed than those who are not in pain.

Researchers note that patients who were depressed before a diagnosis of cancer report more intense pain than those who were not depressed before learning of their disease. Some research also suggests that people with cancer who are also depressed recover more slowly from their illness.

Depression should not be considered an acceptable or inevitable side effect of pain. It can be treated effectively with medication, counseling, or a combination of both. Antidepressant medications are prescribed by psychiatrists, primary care doctors, or oncologists. Effective treatment can help improve an individual's ability to cope with cancer, improve mobility, and even increase decision-making abilities.

The symptoms of clinical depression are listed on the next page. When someone's sad mood lasts more than two weeks or interferes with the ability to carry on day-to-day activities, there is reason for concern. If the help of a trained counselor or therapist is needed, the doctor or nurse will find a therapist who can help people with chronic illnesses such as cancer.

About Depression

What to Look for:
- Persistent sad or "empty" mood almost every day for most of the day.
- Loss of interest or pleasure in ordinary activities.
- Eating problems (loss of appetite or overeating), or significant weight loss or gain.
- Sleep disturbances (insomnia, early waking, or oversleeping).
- Noticeable restlessness or being "slowed down" almost every day.
- Decreased energy, or fatigue almost every day.
- Feelings of guilt, worthlessness, helplessness.
- Difficulty concentrating, remembering, making decisions.
- Thoughts of death or suicide, or attempts at suicide.

Clinical depression is diagnosed if the person has either of the first two symptoms along with at least one of the other symptoms during a two-week period.

What to Do:
- Talk with your doctor about your depression and the possible ways to treat it.
- Seek help through counseling and support groups.
- Increase the amount of contact you have with other people.
- Schedule activities that are pleasant.
- Use prayer or other types of spiritual support.
- Use a problem-solving approach to tackle some of the day-to-day problems that are contributing to your feelings of depression.

Do Not:
- Keep feelings inside—if pain is causing your depression, talk about it.
- Blame yourself for feelings of depression.

Call the Doctor:
- If you have thoughts of suicide.
- If you cannot eat or sleep and feel uninterested in activities of daily living for several days.
- If nothing you do seems to help, even those strategies that have worked in the past.
- If you persistently feel unable to enjoy anything.

Anxiety is an emotional response to fear. Anxiety and fear are common feelings that people with cancer may have. These feelings are normal responses to unpleasant and stressful situations, like pain. Anxiety also may be caused by changes in family roles and responsibilities, loss of control over events in life, changes in body image, uncertainty about the future, and concerns about suffering, pain, and the unknown.

Some people may not always be able to identify their own feelings of anxiety. They may think they are just worried. Before they realize what is happening, they feel out of control. Sometimes a person may become so anxious that he or she may no longer cope well with day-to-day life. If this happens, it may be a good idea to seek help outside the family. Ask your doctor or nurse about your symptoms of anxiety. An assessment can be made to determine whether the side effects of the disease or treatments may be causing the anxiety. Changes in treatment, antianxiety medication, or counseling may be needed.

The Impact of Pain on Relationships

For friends, family members, and caregivers, pain may be one of the most challenging aspects of cancer. It is difficult to watch a person we care for in pain. Caregivers sometimes feel helpless, which leads to feelings of inadequacy and even anger. However, caregivers can greatly influence a person's pain experience by offering their support, both physically and emotionally. The outlook of friends and family can have a significant impact on a patient's attitude about pain relief. If caregivers believe that pain can be relieved, the patient is more likely to believe it too.

People often tolerate pain better when they have enough support and do not feel isolated or like a burden to others. But when social support and human contact is minimal or non-existent, the same person may feel isolated and experience more pain. People whose pain becomes severe enough to prevent them from working will feel even more helpless and isolated.

According to researchers, people with cancer who tap into a solid network of friends and family tolerate pain better than those who confront their pain alone. This support, in fact, may play a critical role in helping people with cancer deal

About Anxiety

What to Look for:
- Feelings of panic.
- Feeling as if you are losing control.
- Difficulty solving problems.
- Feeling excitable.
- Anger or irritation.
- Increased muscle tension.
- Trembling and shaking.
- Headaches, upset stomach, diarrhea, constipation.
- Sweaty palms, racing pulse, difficulty breathing.

What to Do:
- Talk with your doctor about your anxiety and the possible ways to treat it.
- Talk about feelings and fears that you or family members may be having.
- If possible, identify the situations that may be adding to the anxiety.
- Solve day-to-day problems that are causing you stress.
- Engage in some pleasant, distracting activities.
- Seek help through counseling and support groups.
- Use prayer or other types of spiritual support.
- Try deep breathing and relaxation exercises several times a day (see Chapter 7).

Do Not:
- Keep feelings inside—if pain is causing your anxiety, talk about it.
- Blame yourself for feelings of anxiety and fear.

Call the Doctor:
- If you have feelings of panic.
- If you are having trouble breathing, are sweating, and feel very restless.
- If you experience trembling, twitching, and feeling "shaky".
- If your heart rate and pulse have rapidly increased.
- If you have problems sleeping several days in a row.

with pain. In one study[4] involving women with recurrent breast or gynecological cancer, researchers found a strong association between increased social activity and decreased pain levels. The study also noted that as pain increased, people's sense of confidence in how they were doing and their ability to socialize decreased.

Cancer and cancer pain can change relationships outside the family as well as those within. Friends may not keep in touch for a variety of reasons. Some people are afraid of the pain and often unknowingly withhold physical affection. Friends and family may withdraw from people who have become unable to participate in previously shared activities, because they do not want to inflict additional pain on them. Discomfort among friends and family may lead to less contact when people in pain most need their support. Having less intimacy may add to an individual's sense of pain, while increasing physical and social contact may help buffer the experience of pain. Some people prefer to face their pain and illness alone, but most need the comfort and support of friends and family.

Family members and friends who assume caregiving responsibilities play important roles for many people with cancer pain. They often give pain medicines and make sure health professionals are informed about and responsive to the person's pain. They also provide help with routine activities, such as cooking, cleaning, and shopping. In addition to helping in practical ways, caregivers can encourage patients, offer emotional support, and share experiences and knowledge learned from major problems faced in their own lives. Friends and family members may offer an opinion on a treatment choice or take care of household chores. The health care team should involve the caregiver and the person with cancer as much as possible in making decisions about treatment.

People with cancer pain who depend on others to care for them may feel guilty, angry, or depressed by their loss of independence. These emotions are normal, but they can cause strain between people with cancer and their caregivers. The person with cancer is dealing not only with the physical effects of the disease and treatments, but also with the psychological and social challenges of living with cancer. Working together and communicating effectively will help everyone.

Caregivers also feel many pressures. The responsibility of caring for a person in pain can become a burden that is both mentally and physically exhausting.

---

[4] T. A. Rummans, et. al., "Quality of Life and Pain in Patients with Recurrent Breast and Gynecologic Cancer," *Psychosomatics*, 39 (1998): 437-445.

Suggestions for Caregivers:

Helping Patients Cope with Feelings About Cancer Pain

- Help the person with cancer deal with the emotional impact of pain. Some people try to deal with pain by pretending that it doesn't exist. That can be harmful, however, if they do things that make the illness worse, such as avoiding treatment or participating in activities that are physically harmful.
- Support the efforts of the person with cancer to live as normal a life as possible.
- Create a climate that encourages communication. Talk about important or sensitive topics in a manner and place that's calm and conducive to open discussion—not in the midst of a crisis or an argument.
- Be available. One of the most important messages you can communicate is, "If you want to talk about this, I'm willing to listen and talk." However, leave the timing up to the person in pain. To the greatest extent possible, the person with cancer should make decisions on what feelings to share and when, how, and with whom to share them. By not pressing the issue, you allow the person to retain control over part of life at a time when things are beyond control.
- Understand that men and women often communicate differently, and make allowances for those differences. Women sometimes express their feelings more openly than men in our society. If you're a male caregiver and the person with cancer is a woman, be aware when she shares feelings. You may find yourself giving advice when she just wants someone to listen and be understanding. If you're a female caregiver and the person with cancer is male, be aware that he may express his feelings differently than you would. Pay special attention when he talks about things that are important to him. It may be helpful to openly discuss differences in how men and women express feelings and how the person wants to be supported.

But, it is possible for family members to learn how to meet their own needs. Caring for a person with cancer may lead to sadness and feelings of anger that they cannot do more. Caregivers may even feel guilty for being angry, though no one can be blamed for the onset of cancer. If unrecognized or ignored, these feelings can compromise their ability to help.

The needs of everyone can only be determined by discussing the matter openly so that expectations are realistic. People with cancer should discuss what they need and want from caregivers and others who are willing to help. Both should be clear about what the patient needs and expects and how much help a caregiver can provide so there is no confusion about roles.

Asking for Help

Cancer is a complicated disease that requires the attention of a variety of specialists, including surgeons, medical oncologists, radiation oncologists, and teams of support staff. A time may come when a person with cancer needs the services of a mental health professional to help confront the psychological, emotional, and social implications of cancer and cancer pain.

Psychosocial support services are provided by clinicians who understand how cancer and cancer pain affects patients and families and how to help them confront difficult issues related to the illness. These professionals include family counselors, psychologists, therapists, social workers, nurses, and chaplains. Counseling is offered for individuals, couples, families, or in a group setting. Making a decision about what is best depends on a number of factors, such as what services are available and their cost. Ask your health care team about the resources available at your hospital. You can also contact the American Cancer Society to find out about sources of support that are available in your community (see Resources).

WHEN TO SEEK COUNSELING

Your own feelings may be the most useful guide for deciding whether to seek counseling. At the beginning of a cancer experience, most people go through a period of turmoil, which includes feelings of anxiety, sadness, and fear about the future. You may have questions about why this has happened to you, the meaning of your life, and your relationship with God. You may feel worried about your job, finances, insurance, and other practical matters. Gradually, as you get through the first stages of treatment, you will find ways to address your concerns. Cancer-related pain may make your decisions and feelings of success more difficult. Close family members or friends can play a major part in helping you figure out how to deal with cancer pain. An objective observer, such as a counselor or therapist, can identify new and effective ways of coping with cancer and cancer pain.

Chronic feelings of hopelessness, anxiety, and fear will deprive you of the energy you need to cope. If you feel very sad or worried much of the time, or are unable to make decisions, a counselor or other mental health professional can usually help. The advantage in talking with a professional is that you can find quicker solutions to the problems than you would by struggling on your own. Your goal will be to gradually feel more in control of the situation and be able to devote yourself to managing your treatment.

Other family members will have their own concerns as a result of your illness. If you are in a relationship, your partner will try to sort out the meaning of your cancer in relation to his or her own life. Sometimes couples have a hard time talking about a cancer diagnosis, usually because of unspoken fears about the future. If a couple can't figure out how to discuss it, they might benefit by speaking with someone outside of their relationship to gain some perspective.

Finding Support

There are many resources available for people with cancer and their families. Support can come from family and friends as well as health care professionals, support groups, or a place of worship. Asking for support is one way you can take control.

You may live alone or feel lonely. If you do not have support from friends and family, you can find it elsewhere. There are others in your community who need your companionship as much as you need theirs. The mutual support of other people with cancer can be a powerful source of comfort.

SUPPORT GROUPS

Most people with cancer and their families can benefit from support to help manage the physical, emotional, and social aspects of cancer and cancer pain. For example, people who join a patient support group can learn new coping skills and expand their social network. People who participate in group therapy often experience less psychological distress and pain compared with people who do not participate.

The purpose of a support group is to help people share their concerns with others and to learn new ways of solving problems. Participants can expect to learn more about the disease itself as well as getting new ideas from others in the same situation. For instance, a woman with breast cancer can learn from other women about how they have managed episodes of pain.

Support groups for people with cancer can be organized in several different ways. Some meet in hospital settings, within a community agency, a family service agency, or even in a patient's home. They vary widely in size and format, as well as duration. Some groups are small, and meet weekly without a scheduled agenda, while others meet monthly and offer information, teach coping skills, help reduce anxiety, and provide a place to share common concerns and emotional support.

Open-ended groups are set up to allow anyone with cancer or their family members to attend, often for an indefinite period of time. Or people might attend during periods when the course of the illness is changing, decisions need to be made about new treatment options, or new family concerns arise.

Closed groups are those in which the same group of people meet for a set period of time. They can be organized for people with the same diagnosis, the same sex, the same stage of disease, or by the kind of treatment people are receiving.

Groups can be organized by professionals or by cancer survivors. Professionals include oncology social workers or nurses, psychologists, psychiatrists, psychiatric nurses, marriage and family therapists, or clergy. Professionals should be licensed in their respective fields and have skills in group "facilitation." This means they will have had training in how to go about setting up a group and how to help members get their needs met. They also know how to deal with group members who tend to monopolize the conversation or with people who are so upset or angry that a group is counterproductive. If a cancer survivor is facilitating a group, that person may or may not be able to accomplish these tasks. Some cancer survivors are very comfortable dealing with difficult behaviors and have had enough life experience to be very effective in a group setting. Others may not or may find themselves getting uncomfortable or overwhelmed by what is being discussed in the group.

Self-Help Groups

Self-help groups are typically run by nonprofessionals who are affected by a particular situation, such as people who have had cancer. People who relate to your experience firsthand often have treatment-related tips that will be helpful to you. They may offer a home remedy that is helpful with managing pain. In groups without family members, patients are free to express exactly how they feel. Family members benefit similarly from sharing their feelings, fears, and anxieties with other families affected by cancer.

Self-help groups also give those recovering or recovered from cancer an opportunity to aid others who have cancer. With some training, many people with cancer who become group leaders, find that it helps them as well. They get an opportunity to become group counselors or facilitators.

Choosing when to participate in a support group is important. Some find the period at initial diagnosis a difficult time to join a support group. The stories that other people with cancer discuss, after months or even years of treatment, can be overwhelming and upsetting. If you try a group, and it doesn't feel right, you may want to try again at another time.

For those who cannot attend meetings or appointments, counseling over the telephone is offered by organizations such as Cancer Care, Inc. (see Resource Guide). Some people like the privacy of online support groups. Chat rooms and message boards, however, are not the best source of cancer information, especially if they are not monitored by trained professionals or experts. Regardless of the group's structure, participants should feel comfortable in the group and with the facilitator. If you have any fears or uncertainties before entering a group, discuss them with the group's facilitator.

INDIVIDUAL THERAPY

Individual psychotherapy or counseling has also been shown to help patients reduce anxiety and depression, both factors that can intensify pain (see Chapter 2). During individual counseling, people meet one-to-one with a counselor or therapist. The counselor's first objective is to determine specific concerns that need to be addressed. Finding out how you have dealt with problems in the past, including what is or is not working now, is useful in knowing how to proceed. The counselor will help you make sure that your greatest needs are considered. You may talk about different ways to approach a situation before acting on your first impulse. Don't become impatient or frustrated if a strategy doesn't seem to work at first. Problem solving requires sometimes complex solutions and progress may come gradually. Your feelings about your situation, your personality, relationships among family members, ability to be flexible and try new things, and the effects of other life events all influence the counseling process. For example, pain may influence your ability to work, which has implications both personally and professionally.

There are many different types of individual therapy. Some types, such as *cognitive therapy*, are directed at changing behavior by addressing the repetitive, negative thoughts that influence actions. With this type of therapy, people learn to re-program harmful internal messages and create positive thoughts to change behavior. Another type of therapy, called *client-centered therapy*, focuses on people's feelings and current experiences. The therapist in this setting encourages people to lead the sessions while providing empathy and support. The goal is to help people help themselves. *Psychodynamic therapy* is a form of therapy that is geared toward changing life-long personality patterns by uncovering the connections between current emotional reactions and early childhood experiences. This is usually longer-term therapy that focuses on the underlying causes of a problem.

FAMILY THERAPY

Because cancer and cancer pain affects all family members, some health care professionals favor family counseling as an ideal way for families to address their anxieties and worries. People with cancer often state that lack of communication in their families is a problem. Changes in responsibilities can cause resentment and anxiety, but some family members may not feel comfortable openly discussing their feelings.

Family therapy focuses on relationship patterns and all family members may be involved in therapy sessions. A counselor involved in this type of therapy acts as a facilitator to help the family or couple communicate their feelings more effectively. Through family counseling, families learn to deal with changes within the family and help members discuss their feelings more comfortably.

The issues described above apply to all families to some degree at different times. These are typical responses of people dealing with cancer in their families. For many of us, change is difficult. Recognizing problems and understanding why you or family members behave in certain ways are important steps in learning how to talk openly and face the difficult realities when one member of the family has cancer.

Is Family Counseling Right for You?

One of the ways to decide whether to seek family counseling is to think about what is happening in your family. Ask yourself some of the following questions:

- Can I talk to my spouse about how I feel?
- Is my spouse or partner able to listen to what I am saying or does it seem to be too painful for them?
- Does it help to talk to my spouse when things are going badly?
- Do we always end up in a fight about how we are reacting?
- Do my children seem worried?
- Do they tell me how they feel?
- Are my children misbehaving more than usual?
- Is it harder to get them to listen?
- Do my children seem sad or lonely?
- Do they seem unable to enjoy being together as a family?
- Are they fighting among themselves more often?
- Are their grades suffering?
- Am I getting more complaints from my child's school?
- Are my children going backwards in their development? (For example, are they having more difficulty separating from you, maintaining toilet training, being unable to play by themselves, or being unusually dependent on you?)
- Is my family able to accept help from others?
- Do I resent that people outside the immediate family seem happy?
- Do I feel angry a lot of the time that others don't have this burden to deal with?
- Are financial or insurance problems interfering with my ability to deal with my family?

A family counselor will understand how the behavior of individuals influences the family as a whole. The problem may be the way family members communicate with one another. Or it may be a lack of understanding among family members about behaviors that are hurtful or get in the way of people receiving support from each other. Sometimes tension in a family will prevent people from understanding each other so the same hurtful behaviors continue. It is often easier for someone outside the family, such as a counselor, to help family members see a situation differently. Once that is accomplished, the family may be more able to support each other, rather than shutting each other out.

CHOOSING A COUNSELOR

The two most important factors to consider when choosing a counselor or therapist are the person's experience in helping people who have cancer and how comfortable you feel with that person. Professionals who work in cancer treatment centers tend to have more knowledge and experience with emotional responses to cancer than those who do not. Experience working with cancer patients is important because it provides counselors with a framework for understanding your reactions and feelings and greater knowledge about how to improve your situation. For example, an experienced counselor knows that patients often become depressed after initial treatment is completed because the medical facility symbolizes safety and action. It feels safe to many people with cancer to be involved in treatment, rather than spending more time away from treatment. Once treatment ends, patients may worry more than when they were engaged in active measures to control the disease. Counselors recognize this as a normal response and help patients deal with their emotions.

Another important factor to consider in selecting a counselor is professional training and credentials. At a minimum, counselors should possess a master's degree in one of the counseling fields, along with appropriate certification or licensure. Counselors usually come from the fields of social work, psychology, psychiatry, psychiatric nursing, or pastoral counseling. While credentials will demonstrate a person's formal education in a chosen field, they ideally should be backed up with experience working with cancer patients. Don't feel shy about asking about a counselor's experience and education. Professionals who are secure in their abilities know that people need the most knowledgeable source of help and should readily provide you with the information you request.

Some people with cancer believe that unless counselors have endured cancer, they will be of little help. While surviving cancer may add to the counselor's expertise, it is not essential. They have valuable experience gained from working with people with cancer. We have all experienced crises and losses as a normal part of life.

Mental Health Professionals

There are a variety of professionals that offer counseling:

Social workers help people with cancer and their families adjust to the practical and emotional problems related to illness. They focus on social functioning, which includes helping people with community and financial resources, health care systems, employment concerns, legal and ethical issues, insurance coverage, child care, and other needs. Oncology social workers specialize in helping people manage concerns related to cancer and work closely with health care professionals who treat people with cancer.

Psychologists are licensed professionals who usually have doctoral degrees (Ph.D., Psy.D., Ed.D.) and provide counseling and psychotherapy, testing if needed, teaching, and consultation. They may also do research. Psycho-oncologists are psychologists who are experienced in counseling people with cancer and their loved ones. They can help people adjust to illness, manage anxiety and depression, and cope with other emotional problems.

Psychiatrists specialize in the field of medicine that focuses on the diagnosis and treatment of mental illness. Psychiatrists are licensed doctors (M.D.s) who can prescribe medication to treat psychiatric illness and conduct psychotherapy.

Marriage and family therapists are mental health professionals trained in couples counseling and family therapy. They are licensed in many states to work with people who have problems in their relationships, marriages, or families. They

Consider how you feel when you first meet with a counselor or therapist. Does it feel safe to share your concerns with this person? Do you trust the counselor's ability to help you? Do you feel that the counselor listens well and understands you as an individual? Do you think your family could relate easily to this person? Trust your instincts. If somehow you just don't feel comfortable after a few sessions, it's probably wise to try someone else. You will know when you have found the right match.

have graduate training (a master's or doctoral degree) in marriage and family therapy and at least two years of clinical experience. If your state does not offer licensure, inquire if the therapist is certified in marriage and family therapy from the American Association of Marriage and Family Therapists (AAMFT).

Licensed professional counselors provide mental health and substance abuse counseling in a variety of settings. They are licensed in many states to work with individuals, families, groups and organizations. They have a master's degree or above and are trained in understanding human growth, development, and psychosocial problems.

Pastoral counselors focus on spiritual beliefs for psychological healing and growth. Certified pastoral counselors have mental health and religious training.

Psychiatric nurses conduct assessments of patients' psychosocial and physical needs; offer assistance with basic life skills; and provide individual, group, and family counseling, training, and education. They are trained and certified as nurses who specialize in mental health services.

You can get referrals by asking members of your health care team, or by contacting professional organizations for names of psychotherapists who specialize in the area. Oncology units of hospitals sometimes have departments that staff counselors.

WHY DO SOME PEOPLE NEED HELP AND OTHERS DON'T?

One of the concerns for people needing support services is how they feel about asking for help. Some people have the idea that they should know how to handle every emotional problem even though they have never been confronted with a crisis like cancer. Sometimes people feel that needing help with a problem is a sign of weakness. This is not true. In fact, asking for help can be a sign of strength. Learning about what you might expect from yourself and other family members can help you solve problems quicker than attempting to solve them alone.

How Will I Know if Counseling is Working

You will know if counseling is helping you and your family if you can answer "yes" to at least some of the following questions:

- Are you gaining more insight into your problems?
- Is it becoming easier to keep the situation in perspective?
- Do you feel like you have more options?
- Do you feel less anxious or worried?
- Has your concentration improved?
- Is it easier to make decisions?
- Do you have a clear idea where you are going or what needs working on immediately and what can wait until later?
- Are you more in control over how you are feeling and behaving?
- Has your performance improved at work or home?
- Can the counselor give you some idea of how long you will need help?
- Can you tell your doctor how counseling is helping?

Ask family members the same questions if they are involved in counseling. If your answers to these questions seem positive, you are probably on the right track. If you don't feel good about your answers to these questions, discuss them with your counselor. If your relationship with the counselor is uncomfortable or lacks trust, it may be that you expect different things from the therapist or that you misunderstand the counseling process in some way. It may also mean that you need to find someone who is a better match for your personality or situation. Finding the right counselor or therapist may take time and effort, but the reward is often great for you and your family.

It is good to ask for help early to prepare for the challenges of treatment. During periods of active treatment, you may be in too much pain or feel too overwhelmed to seek help. In addition to your physical needs, family members will have their own reactions and worries. If you are experiencing a great deal of pain, it may be harder for you to feel in charge of the situation. By enlisting help early in the process, you can focus more energy on your treatment for cancer or pain.

For some people, the idea of getting professional help for emotional or family problems is not acceptable. They feel that somehow needing help means that they are "weak" or a sign that they are unstable or even "crazy." It may seem to you that some people sail through the cancer experience, without outward signs of stress. People make judgments about themselves and say things like "what's wrong with me that I cannot seem to cope with my problems?" Or, "I should be able to just 'tough it out' until the trouble passes." While we all sometimes feel as if we should be able to manage just about anything, there will be times in this experience that telling yourself to be strong just does not work.

Learning what you need to know about cancer medically along with what you can expect of yourself and your family takes time. Sorting through the medical aspects of cancer is an enormous challenge in itself. People with cancer may not have the energy to cope alone with the added burden of emotional issues. They may get ignored until life feels more settled. This is understandable, since people can only cope with so much at one time. Struggling alone is unnecessary. Asking for help in understanding and anticipating what is to come is best for you and your family. Give yourself the benefit of other people's experiences and insights so that you can approach the situation with as much hope and optimism as possible. That way you can manage your illness, and get on with your life.

Realize that it may not be possible to control everything going on in your life. Having cancer or cancer-related pain is new territory and it will take some time to discover what strategies work best for you. Don't be hesitant or afraid to seek the support you need in order to feel better.

WILL INSURANCE PAY FOR COUNSELING AND THERAPY SERVICES?

Insurance benefits for counseling services depend on your particular health plan and its coverage for mental health services. Most health plans offer at least some coverage for counseling, but often it is limited. Some policies only pay for a few counseling or psychotherapy sessions, or they may limit your choices of which professionals you can visit. Your insurance company may have contracts that obligate it to use certain mental health providers. If you don't understand your coverage, ask a hospital or clinic social worker for help. If counseling services are not available free of charge where you receive cancer treatment, a social worker can usually help you find accurate information about your plan and what is covered. A hospital's billing department may also examine your policy and determine your coverage. Social workers often know about services in the community that adjust their fees according to your income. Some hospitals and community health centers even offer free counseling or support groups.

Chapter 9

Dealing with the Financial Burden of Cancer Treatment

"No question is too small or too silly to ask. I was never afraid to call the doctor or staff with questions about anything—even questions about our bills and insurance. I found that our doctor and his staff were willing to answer any question. It was also very helpful to speak with our pharmacist. He made special arrangements when we needed to get prescriptions, especially pain medicine, filled after regular business hours."

Judith, a caregiver for her husband

The costs related to cancer treatment can be substantial, leading to significant financial pressures for patients and their families. The financial impact of cancer may be magnified by the potential lost days of work and income during a patient's treatment and recovery. People with cancer may have to rely entirely on the income of a spouse or partner. For single patients or those whose spouses are unable to work, the financial stress is even greater. This stress on families compounds the emotional distress caused by cancer, creating yet another source of anxiety for patients and their families as medical bills accumulate.

Insurance coverage for cancer diagnosis and treatment varies widely. Some health plans provide extensive coverage, while others offer minimal or no coverage. Coverage for prescription medicines is even less predictable. For the uninsured, the financial demands may be extreme, stretching patients and their families to their financial limits and often putting families deep into debt.

Workplace health benefits, when they are offered to employees, also vary considerably. But, a number of laws protect employees who experience a serious illness and who must take extended absences from their jobs.

During treatment, most of a family's focus is on treating the disease and on the physical and emotional well being of the person with cancer. Yet even during these difficult times, patients and their families need to turn at least some of their attention to the financial aspects of dealing with cancer.

Taking Stock of Your Financial Situation

You need to know where you stand financially before you can take actions to improve your position. Are medical bills still coming in? How much debt has accumulated? Will you have a regular paycheck soon to help pay expenses? How do you rebuild your accounts? These are not easy questions, and you may not want to face a financial problem because it is yet another source of strain during a time of emotional upheaval and physical discomfort or pain. Still, taking stock of your finances is an important step in taking back control of your life.

SOURCES OF FINANCIAL HELP

During and after treatment, many people find themselves struggling with financial problems. While you're regaining your physical strength, you may also need to work on getting your finances in order. A case manager or a financial planner may be helpful in guiding you through the often-complicated process of assessing and improving your financial situation.

Even if health insurance pays for most of your costs, out-of-pocket expenses can still be a major financial burden. If you've found gaps in your coverage, don't hesitate to discuss your needs with your doctor or hospital social worker. The number of organizations that exist to help you and other people with cancer may surprise you.

Keep in mind that your hospital social worker can refer you to organizations that provide lodging for people undergoing treatment and their families. The American Cancer Society (ACS) offers this service in some locations as well (call 800-ACS-2345 for information about Hope Lodges). Your hospital social worker can also refer you to organizations that provide free or reduced transportation, airfare, and other resources.

Financial Resources

You have several options for getting assistance with financial problems. Possible sources of help and relief for families in financial need include:

- Income assistance for low-income families through Supplemental Security Insurance (SSI) benefits.
- Income assistance for non-working parents from the Aid to Families with Dependent Children (AFDC) program.
- Help with travel, meals, and lodging from public and private programs.
- Assistance with basic living costs (rent, mortgage, insurance premiums, utilities, telephone) from public and private programs.
- Help from church, civic, social, and fraternal groups in the community.
- General help from special funds in the medical center or community.
- Assistance from targeted fundraising for an individual patient or family.
- Low-interest loans from family or friends.
- Medication assistance programs.
- Home equity conversion.
- Declaration of bankruptcy.

Your hospital social worker or a financial assistance planner can be helpful in guiding you through the often-complicated process of accessing financial resources.

PAYING YOUR BILLS

You may have difficulty keeping up with the direct and indirect costs of treatment as well as the regular expenses of daily life. The easiest way to face money problems is to approach them one step at a time. You can set up payment plans with utility providers, mortgage or rental managers, doctors, and other medical providers. If you have a good history of paying your bills on time, most businesses and creditors will probably allow you to arrange a payment plan.

Because many out-of-pocket expenses aren't covered by insurance, people often use credit cards to pay for expenses during cancer treatment. It is common for people to find that their credit card debt quickly becomes unmanageable.

Suggestions for Managing Your Financial Situation

- Become familiar with your individual insurance plan and its provisions. If additional insurance is needed, learn through your carrier whether it is available to you.
- Submit claims for all medical expenses, even when you are uncertain about your coverage.
- Keep accurate and complete records of claims submitted, pending, and paid so you know when you have reached the reimbursement limit.
- Keep copies of documentation related to your claims, such as letters of medical necessity, bills, receipts, requests for sick leave, and correspondence with insurance companies.
- In times of strained finances, enlist the help of a caseworker, a hospital financial counselor, or a social worker. Often, payment arrangements can be made if companies or hospitals are aware of your situation.
- Submit your bills as you receive them. If you become overwhelmed with bills, get help.
- Contact local support organizations, such as your American Cancer Society or your state government agencies, for information on other resources.
- Do not allow insurance to expire. Pay premiums in full and on time. It is often difficult to get new insurance.

One temporary solution is to consolidate all credit card balances to the card that charges the lowest interest rates. Making small but consistent payments is better than making no payments at all. If you can't meet the minimum payments, call the credit card company. If you explain your situation, the company will usually try to make arrangements with you. They would rather that you make some attempt to pay than not pay at all. It's also possible to negotiate for lower interest rates.

Credit counseling agencies can offer assistance dealing with credit worries. The Consumer Credit Counseling Service is a national nonprofit service that offers free and confidential financial counseling. They help people set up budgets and make repayment plans. Their counselors are certified and often offer appointments on a same-day basis. Your local Consumer Credit Counseling office is listed in the business section of the *White Pages*. You can also call their toll-free number at 800-251-2227 to schedule a telephone or in-person session. Additionally, they offer credit counseling on the Internet (http://www.cccsatl.org/online.html).

If your financial situation is complex, or if you feel overwhelmed by the financial burden imposed by cancer and cancer treatment, consider seeking the help of a professional financial advisor. Make sure the advisor you choose has experience handling finances associated with a serious illness.

To answer legal questions, consult an attorney who specializes in areas such as insurance law, estate planning, or discrimination in employment. This advice may be available free of charge at a legal counseling center in your area.

Health Insurance

PRIVATE INSURANCE

Many patients are covered by private insurance through employee group plans or individual plans. These insurance plans are offered in several forms and a range of payment plans and models. The more services covered by the policy, the higher the premiums. Some private insurance plans pay for prescription medications, others may not. Prescription medication coverage is particularly

Money Matters

A good resource to consider when getting your finances in order is the *Taking Charge of Money Matters* workshop and pamphlet offered by the American Cancer Society's I CAN COPE program. This series offers financial guidance for cancer survivors and their families. Topics include the fundamentals of insurance, estate planning, returning to work, disability insurance, how to improve your financial planning, financial resources, and how to create a budget. Call 800-ACS-2345 to learn more about this program and booklet series.

helpful for patients taking medications for pain, since a great deal of pain treatment involves prescription medications.

Over the past several years, the health insurance industry has been transformed. In many regions of the country, traditional policies (in which patients can choose the medical professionals that treat them) have been replaced by some form of managed care, which includes health maintenance organizations (HMOs) and preferred provider organizations (PPOs). Managed care is designed to provide comprehensive health care for patients by member doctors and specialists associated with particular plans. Patients generally pay lower premiums than they would for traditional health insurance, but they are somewhat restricted in the choices they can make about their medical treatment. Enrollment is usually offered when you are first hired, and/or during a specific time each year, called open enrollment. At these times, applicants are generally accepted for coverage regardless of health history or pre-existing conditions.

You need to be aware of your coverage and your rights in order to deal with any insurance issues that arise. Many managed care plans pay the costs for prescription medications, including pain relief medications, but the insurer controls the type, amount, and even the brand of prescription medications. Managed care organizations often require members to pay a small deductible or copayment when they receive services or medications. Read your insurance policy carefully to determine what treatment services and medications it covers. If you find that your policy is difficult to interpret, contact a representative from your insurance company for clarification. A hospital social worker may also be able to help you sort things out.

If you have health insurance through your employer and you are considering leaving your job, don't do so until you have explored health insurance conversion options. Many employee health plans have a clause that allows for conversion to individual plans, although premiums may be considerably higher. These individual plans usually must be applied for within thirty days of termination.

If you consider converting your insurance coverage from an employee plan, be aware of differences in coverage. Ask about choices of physicians, protection against cancellations, and increases in premiums. Determine what the plan really covers, especially in the event of catastrophic illness. Ask about deductibles and the maximum lifetime coverage amount. Remember that the more comprehensive the insurance policy, the higher are the deductibles and copayments.

Questions to Ask About Your Insurance

You may want to ask your insurance agent the following questions as you evaluate your options.

What does my insurance cover?

- Is there a toll-free number I can call to get information? Is it important to speak to the same person each time I call?
- Does my policy have a monetary limit on benefits?
- Will my hospital stay be covered?
- How do I find out if a procedure is covered? Who do I call?
- If I want to see a doctor who is out of network, will that be covered?
- Are the costs of participating in a clinical trial covered?
- Does my policy cover all my expenses through several rounds of chemotherapy or radiation?
- Does my policy cover recurrence and subsequent treatment?
- Does my policy cover breast reconstruction after a mastectomy?
- Which breast cancer treatments are covered under this policy?
- Does my policy cover implant surgery, including the implant, anesthesia, and other hospital costs?
- Does my policy cover treatments for medical problems that may result from the implant or reconstruction?
- Does my policy cover the removal of implants?
- If I wait to have my breast reconstructed, will the reconstruction still be covered under my policy?

What about additional coverage and out-of-pocket expenses?

- Is there any way I can appeal for additional coverage if I need it?
- What will I have to pay out of pocket?
- What programs are available to help me with the costs of traveling to and from treatment centers?
- How much can the government help me?
- Do I qualify for any special benefits?
- Can I claim any of these expenses on my taxes?

THE CONSOLIDATED OMNIBUS BUDGET
RECONCILIATION ACT (COBRA)

This law, passed in 1986, allows employees to keep their health plans after leaving a job. It is effective only if you had a health plan at work, and it must be applied for within sixty days after your employment ends. An employer has the obligation to notify an employee in writing of COBRA's availability and options. Continuing insurance coverage is available if the premium is paid on schedule and until the individual becomes covered under another group or individual policy. Under COBRA, you can keep your old health plan for up to eighteen months. If you qualify as disabled, the coverage lasts up to twenty-nine months, and in some circumstances, dependents may be covered up to thirty-six months. However, the premiums are likely to be higher because you become responsible for paying the entire amount.

Finding out if you qualify for COBRA serves two purposes. First, it can extend your health care coverage. Second, it can help you qualify for a private health care policy. For example, if you use COBRA to maintain your employer's health insurance coverage after leaving your job, you cannot be turned down for insurance even if you have a pre-existing condition. The program is administered by the U.S. Department of Labor, which can provide you with detailed information about the program (see Resources).

THE HEALTH INSURANCE PORTABILITY AND
ACCOUNTABILITY ACT (HIPAA)

This law, passed in 1996, provides nationwide standards and a guarantee of access to health insurance coverage for individuals. This legislation protects people from discrimination based on pre-existing medical conditions. Because of this, many employees don't lose their insurance when they change jobs or move to a different state.

HIPPA includes several provisions that may benefit parents of children or adolescents with cancer. It enables a parent who has had group medical insurance for at least twelve months to change jobs and be guaranteed other coverage with a new employer who also offers group insurance. There is no waiting period and an individual or dependent cannot be denied coverage because of a pre-existing health problem. If a parent was previously uninsured and takes a job with an employer offering group insurance, the waiting period for individuals with pre-existing conditions cannot be longer than twelve months. The plan also requires insurers to renew coverage to all employers and individuals when premiums are paid, and it guarantees availability of group insurance coverage for businesses that employ two to fifty people. For more information about HIPAA, contact your state department or commission of insurance.

INSURANCE FROM PROFESSIONAL ORGANIZATIONS

As a cancer patient, group coverage may be your only option. You may be able to get insurance through trade, alumni, or professional organizations such as those for retired persons, teachers, social workers, realtors, etc. Most of these require proof of insurability. Look for a "guaranteed issue" plan, which is a plan where employees are eligible for benefits regardless of prior health history. Also, check to make sure that any non-employer group plan is allowed in your state.

DISABILITY INSURANCE

Some health insurance policies include long-term disability protection, which typically pays 60 to 70 percent of your monthly income if you are unable to work. (The amount of your income has nothing to do with whether you qualify for benefits.) Most disability policies contain a pre-existing condition exclusion period. If you pay the cost of this insurance yourself, the benefits will be income tax free. If your employer pays the cost of this insurance, the benefits are taxable. Disability plans can be either short-term or long-term. If you have to stop work for over a month, find out if you have a long-term disability insurance policy through your place of employment.

PAYING FOR MEDICATIONS NOT COVERED BY INSURANCE

If your insurance plan does not pay for prescription medications used to relieve pain, you can try other sources of help, such as one of the drug assistance programs listed by the Pharmaceutical Research and Manufacturers of America (PhRMA; see Resources). PhRMA offers information about pharmaceutical companies and drugs that are currently available, in clinical trials, or under development. The web site includes a directory of patient assistance programs for prescription drugs and a database of new medications for cancer and other diseases. Also, talk with your doctor or pharmacist about less expensive drugs or generic forms that may be available.

You may not have any trouble getting claims covered by your insurance company, but if a claim is denied at any time, ask for help from your doctor's office or from the hospital claims office. Sometimes an insurance company denies claims based on specific language in the policy. To figure out if the denial is due to an interpretation of the policy, ask the company for the exact language that supports the coverage denial. To find out about the appeal process for disputed claims, call your insurance company.

If you feel you have been treated unfairly by a private insurance company or HMO, contact your state insurance commission. State insurance commissions monitor insurance companies and can force them to pay restitution to policyholders if needed. Complaint forms are available on web sites of many state insurance departments, which may be willing to work with your health care providers and insurance company to help get coverage for procedures, services, or medications that are denied. For more information, visit the National Association of Insurance Commissioner's web site at http://www.naic.org.

If a Claim is Denied

Sometimes insurers deny particular claims to pay for tests, procedures, medications, or other services ordered by a doctor. If this occurs, it is important to have a good working relationship with a customer service representative or case manager at your insurance company with whom the situation can be discussed. A first step should be to resubmit the claim, accompanied by a copy of the denial letter. If the patient is a child, the child's doctor may be required to explain or justify what has been done or requested. Sometimes the test or service simply needs to be "coded" differently. If questioning or challenging the denial in these ways is not successful, then families may need to:

- Postpone payment until the matter is resolved.
- Resubmit the claim a third time and request a review.
- Ask to speak with a supervisor who may have authority to reverse a decision.

If you'd like to file a complaint about a federal qualified HMO, contact the U.S. Health Care Financing Administration. If you need help filing a claim related to a private employer, union self-insurance, or self-financed plan, contact the U.S. Department of Labor, Pension, and Welfare Benefits Administration (see Resources).

Medicaid complaints may be directed to the state department of social services or medical assistance services, while Medicare complaints may be filed with the U.S. Social Security Administration (see Resources). Disputes regarding veterans' benefits are handled through the U.S. Department of Veterans Affairs (800-733-8387).

You can also get more information from the Health Insurance Association of America (HIAA). They represent most health insurance companies in the United States. Their web site contains insurance guides and general insurance information, and an annual directory and survey of hospitals, along with other information (see Resources).

- Formally appeal the denial in writing, explaining why you think the claim should be paid. Your health care team members may be able to help with this.
- Request a written response.
- Keep all originals of correspondence in your possession. Your health care team may be able to help you make copies if necessary.
- Keep a record of dates, names, and conversations you have about the denial.
- Seek help from the consumer services division of your state insurance department or commission.
- Ask for help from the Candlelighter's Foundation ombudsman program (see Resources).
- Be persistent in trying to resolve the matter.
- Consider legal action.

Government Sources of
Health Insurance and Assistance

MEDICARE

Medicare is a program of the federal government that is funded by the Social Security Administration. It provides health insurance for retired people who are at least sixty-five years old, those who have been disabled for more than two years, or those who have received Social Security disability benefits for at least twenty-four months. Many doctors and hospitals accept Medicare payment. HMOs that have contracts with Medicare must provide all hospital and medical benefits covered by the program. However, you must usually obtain services from the HMO's network of health care providers. Medicare provides basic health coverage, but it doesn't pay all medical expenses.

Medicare is divided into two parts. Part A provides benefits for hospital care, home health care, hospice care, and care in Medicare-certified nursing facilities. Part B, which is paid separately by the individual, covers diagnostic studies, physician services, durable medical equipment used at home, and ambulance transportation.

Generally, Medicare only pays for the costs of medications that are given during a hospital stay. This lack of coverage for prescription medications is a major reason why many people consider purchasing additional Medicare insurance policies to fill in the gaps not covered by the original policy. These policies are called Medigap or Medicare Supplemental Insurance.

MEDICAID

Medicaid is a program jointly sponsored by the federal government and individual states. The plan covers low-income patients who are either elderly, blind, disabled, or have dependent children, and pregnant women whose income is below the family poverty level.

Each state has an agency that administers Medicaid and sets regulations concerning Medicaid use and what income levels qualify people for benefits. Benefits, rules, and regulations vary from state to state and are often complex. Eligibility is determined by specialists in county departments of social services or welfare. Not all doctors and hospitals accept Medicaid patients.

Unlike Medicare, Medicaid pays for many prescription medications. Many Medicaid plans cover medications given at doctors' offices as well as pain medications taken at home. However, depending on the state, there may be limits on the amount of medications the plan will pay for. Families with an income low enough to qualify for Medicaid may also receive special consideration or classification by hospitals and medical centers that could result in a discounted bill.

In some situations, Medicaid will pay for nonmedical expenses, such as food, lodging, and the cost of transportation to hospitals and clinics if a parent has to travel out of the community for a child's treatment or follow-up care. For detailed information about Medicaid, contact your state's Medicaid office.

BENEFITS FOR VETERANS AND THEIR FAMILIES

Veterans qualify for significant health benefits from the government. However, veterans' benefits are changing and the number of veterans' medical facilities is declining. To get the most accurate information, call the Department of Veteran Affairs at 800-733-8387.

TRICARE (formerly CHAMPUS) is a federal program that helps pay for the civilian medical care of dependents of active-duty, retired, or deceased members of the armed services. Benefits include skilled nursing care, professional medical home-care services, social work services, counseling, medications, and medical supplies and equipment. Information about TRICARE coverage is available from the Benefits Advisor at the nearest military medical facility (see Resources).

HILL-BURTON PROGRAM

A number of hospitals and other medical facilities receive funds from the federal government so they can offer free or low-cost services to those who are unable to pay. This is called the Hill-Burton Program. Each facility chooses which services it will provide free or at lowered cost. People covered by Medicare and Medicaid are not eligible for this coverage. However, Hill-Burton may cover services not covered by other government programs. Eligibility for this plan is based on family size and income. You may apply for this assistance at any time, before or after you receive care (see Resources).

SOCIAL SECURITY DISABILITY INCOME (SSDI)

This government program pays benefits if you are disabled. You must meet Social Security's strict definition of disability, which is narrow. If you get turned down the first time you apply, you may be approved if you reapply. Some cases that are originally turned down are approved after an appeal. If approved, benefits do not begin until the sixth month of disability. Also, you must have paid the minimum amount into the Social Security fund and worked at least five of the last ten years. For contact information see Resources section at the back of this book.

SUPPLEMENTAL SECURITY INCOME (SSI)

If you have not worked much or if your income was very low before you were able to return to work, you may be eligible for SSI. To qualify, your income and assets must fall below a certain level and you must be disabled, over sixty-five, and/or blind. The amount of benefits you receive varies from state to state. If you do qualify, you could receive as much as $500 per month. More information about SSI can be obtained from your social worker or from the nearest Social Security Administration office listed in the U.S. Government section of the telephone book.

AID TO FAMILIES WITH DEPENDENT CHILDREN (AFDC)

AFDC is a state and federally funded program administered by each state department of social services or welfare. It provides financial assistance to eligible families. AFDC recipients are also eligible for Medicaid. For more information contact your county department of social services or welfare.

CHILDREN'S SPECIAL HEALTH SERVICES (CSHS)

CSHS is a state-administered program providing financial support for individuals twenty-one years of age and younger who have certain chronic conditions, including cancer. It is financed by both state and federal funds. In some states, these programs may have different names. For more information about whether you can benefit from this program, consult with a hospital financial counselor or talk with your social worker.

Other Financial Resources and Options

The following health care resources may be available to help you pay for medical services and medications.

Government Sources of Health Care Coverage

Sources of Health Care Coverage	Issues
Medical Insurance	Must continue paying premiums.
COBRA	18–36 month extension of group health benefits. Must pay premium.
Hill-Burton Program (low-cost or no-cost health care)	Must use Hill-Burton facilities Not all services are available. Eligibility based on family size and income (income below current poverty guidelines).
Medicare	Eligibility based on same criteria as Social Security benefits or Railroad retirement benefits and certain other health problems. Must pay for part B of program.
Medicaid (contact state office)	Eligibility based on family size, assets, and income.
Veteran's Benefits (contact local office)	Service-connected problems are generally covered. May require low income for certain benefits. May require some deductibles.

MEDICAL ASSISTANCE PROGRAMS

Medical assistance programs are available in states for those with incomes under certain amounts. The scope of these programs varies from state to state, but they may provide money for expenses such as prescription medications, doctors' visits, hospitalizations, and insurance premiums. A hospital social worker or case manager in your area should be able to provide more information about these local programs. Check into the renewal requirements as you investigate this option so that you'll be prepared if quarterly renewal is required.

OPTIONS FOR THE UNINSURED

If you get turned down for a private policy, you may be eligible for a state-sponsored plan. These plans were designed to provide health care coverage for hard-to-insure people. The cost of a state plan will be high, but at least you will have health coverage.

A number of states currently sell comprehensive health insurance to state residents with serious medical conditions who can't find a company to insure them. These state programs (sometimes called risk pools), serve people who have pre-existing health conditions and who are often denied or have difficulty finding affordable coverage in the private market.

Risk Pools

Health insurance risk pools (also called guaranteed access programs) are special programs created by state legislatures to provide a safety net for the "medically uninsurable" population. These people have been denied health insurance coverage because of a pre-existing health condition or can only access private coverage that is restricted or has extremely high rates.

Each state risk pool is different. Generally, each program operates as a state developed nonprofit association overseen by a board of directors made up of industry, consumer, and state insurance department representatives. The board contracts with an established insurance company to collect premiums, pay claims, and administrate the program on a day-to-day basis. Insurance benefits vary, but risk pools typically offer benefits that are comparable to basic private market plans. Maximum lifetime benefits also vary by state, ranging from as low as $250,000 to $1 million (some even have no upper limit).

Group plan issuers who participate in state risk pools may deny, exclude, or limit an enrollee's benefits arising from a pre-existing condition for a waiting period of no more than twelve months following the effective date of coverage. Without this waiting period, the concern is that too many people could file high-cost claims before paying any insurance, making the program unable to function financially. However, some states waive waiting periods for people who show they have had continual coverage in the private market. Risk pool insurance generally

Additional Financial Resources

Sources of Health Care Coverage	Issues
Disability Income Insurance	Must pay premiums until waived by insurance company. May affect qualifying for government benefits. Must meet definition of disability under policy.
Reverse Mortgage	Creates income tax obligation. May affect qualifying for some government benefits. May ultimately require payments. Must pass credit check. Some age restrictions.
Social Security	Must be disabled or retired. May create income tax obligation. May affect qualifying for other government benefits.
SSI (Supplemental Security Income)	Must be disabled, over age 65, and/or blind. Must meet income restrictions. May affect qualifying for other government benefits.
Temporary Aid to Needy Families	Must meet low-income guidelines. May require disability. May require employment history.

costs more than standard insurance, but laws in each state set a cap on premiums to protect individuals from exorbitant costs.

Risk pools aren't meant to serve the indigent or poor who cannot afford health insurance; they are designed to serve people who would not otherwise have the right to purchase health insurance protection. The indigent can access coverage through state medical assistance, Medicaid, or similar programs. However, some state risk pools do have a subsidy for lower-income, medically uninsurable people.

Independent Brokers

An independent broker may be able to help you locate a reasonable benefit package. Group insurance is usually preferable to individual insurance.

OTHER ORGANIZATIONS

Civic and religious organizations may offer financial help or services for people with cancer and their family members. Groups such as the Salvation Army, United Way, Lutheran Social Services, and Catholic Social Services are listed in the Yellow Pages under "Social Service Organizations." Churches and synagogues may also be able to help with transportation, baby-sitting, and home-care services. The Federal Consumer Information Center offers information about managing debt and many other topics. You can call them toll free at 800-688-9889 or 800-326-2996 (TDD), or visit their web site at http://www.pueblo.gsa.gov. Call your American Cancer Society at 1-800-ACS-2345 or your local unit for information on services and resources in your community.

HOME EQUITY CONVERSION

You may be able to convert part of your home's equity into cash if you are at least sixty-two years old and own your home (or nearly own it). The most common type of equity conversion is called a "reverse mortgage." This is a loan against your home that doesn't have to be repaid for as long as you live there. The loan is repaid in the future—usually when the last surviving borrower sells, dies, or moves out of the home. It can provide cash to pay medical bills and other expenses, but it is still considered a loan and includes expenses such as interest charges and service fees. A reverse mortgage can also disqualify you from some government programs. Private, public, and federally insured lenders offer many types of reverse mortgage programs. Contact a financial advisor to find out if a reverse mortgage would help you (see National Association of Personal Financial Advisors in Resources section at the back of this book).

You can also get more information about home equity conversion from non-profit consumer groups, such as the American Association of Retired Persons (AARP; see Resources).

RETIREMENT PLANS

Some people use money from their retirement plan as a source of cash before they retire. You may qualify for hardship provisions so that you don't pay any penalties for early withdrawal of money. Contact a financial advisor or the human resources office at your place of employment for more information.

FAMILY LOANS

Family members may be willing to pay for some of your medication costs or other cancer-related expenses. If you ask for a loan from a relative, outline a repayment period and an interest rate. (Keep in mind that there are federal tax consequences if the person making the loan charges you an interest rate below the minimum federal rate.) To protect all parties and avoid misunderstandings, put the agreement in writing. Tax laws in this area are complicated, so it's a good idea to consult an accountant about family loans.

If you don't think you will be able to repay the loan, ask for a gift instead. Anyone, including a relative, can give a gift of up to $10,000 each year, which is tax-free to the recipient. Married couples can give a gift of up to $20,000 per year tax-free to the recipient. Any gifts over these limits are considered taxable income. (The gifts do not provide tax deductions to the person offering the gift.) Also, anyone can pay the medical bills of someone else without being subject to the gift limit, if the payment is made directly to the medical facility.

LIFE INSURANCE

The amount of life insurance you need depends on your unique situation. A financial advisor can help you decide how much life insurance is enough. Some employers offer life insurance as a benefit. For example, you may be offered life insurance equal to one or two times your yearly income. Some employers pay the entire cost of this insurance. You may be able to buy additional life insurance and pay for it yourself. But any additional coverage you buy may require proof of insurability.

For someone who has recently gone through cancer treatment, the only type of life insurance available may be "guaranteed" or "simplified issue." With this kind of insurance, very few questions are asked about your health. However, the cost of the policy is usually high. These policies also may set limits before they would pay a death benefit. For example, some policies say that if you die within two years of buying the policy, your heirs would not receive the benefit. The only money they would get is the amount you paid into premiums, plus interest. If you die after the two-year period, the death benefit would be paid. If you are a long-term cancer survivor, you may be able to purchase a more typical form of life insurance, though not all companies will insure someone with a cancer history. You may have to look at several companies before you find one that

Sources of Cash

As you consider sources of cash, make sure you recognize the issues involved with the liquidation or sale of each asset listed below. Consider implications such as tax obligations and permanent repercussions on your estate.

Sources of Lump-Sum Cash	Issues
Assets (sale of stock, real estate, etc.)	May create income tax obligation. May affect qualifying for government benefits.
Home Equity Loan (may be lump sum or line of credit)	Puts home at risk. Must have equity in home. Must make regular payments. Must pass credit check.
Family/Personal Loan	Requires repayment. May strain family relationships. May require collateral.

meets your needs. A good insurance agent can help you find a company that specializes in hard-to-insure individuals.

Viaticals

Life-threatening illnesses and conditions requiring extensive medical care often require immediate financial resources. In many states, the value of an individual's life insurance policy can be realized through the acceleration of the policy's death benefit—known as "living benefits." These benefits can be accessed several ways, including a viatical (sale of the life insurance policy) and loans from the original insurance company or a third party against the face value of the life insurance policy.

Policy Loan (from life insurance company)	Death benefit is reduced by the amount of the loan and accrued interest. Must have "cash value" type of policy. Must generally continue premium payments.
Accelerated Death Benefits (life insurance)	Must keep policy in force. Must be terminally ill (contact insurance company). May create income tax obligation. May affect qualifying for government benefits.
Viatical Loan (borrow from investor using life insurance as collateral) *or* Viatical Settlement (sell life insurance policy to investor)	May create income tax obligation. Must own policy. Must meet definition of terminally or chronically ill. May affect qualifying for government benefits.

Before Signing a Contract for a Viatical or Living Benefits

Before you make a final decision about selling your life insurance policy, consider the points below. Talk to a lawyer or a financial planner to help you decide what might be best for your situation.

- Get a clear picture of what's involved. Read about viaticals.
- Get professional advice regarding types of living benefits available and their positives and negatives.
- Decide whether a viatical is really the best course of action for you.
- Attempt to verify life expectancy.
- Find out if Medicaid or other benefits will be affected.
- Shop around. Get several bids. Bids can vary from 35 to 80 percent of the policy.
- Find out if the company is a broker. Some companies use their own money to buy policies, but others are brokers. A broker gets a commission from the company and may not act in the best interest of the insured.
- Negotiate to get the best deal you can.

A viatical is the sale of a life insurance policy for cash, which is used to pay for daily living expenses, medical care, or other pressing needs. The process of selling a life insurance policy requires the person insured for a life-threatening illness to sell his or her life insurance policy to a third party.

A viatical insurance company buys policies from people with terminal illnesses. After the viatical company buys a policy, the company becomes the new owner and sole beneficiary of the policy. It pays the premiums on the policy as long as the patient is alive. When the person dies, all the remaining money from the policy goes to the viatical company. A viatical transaction usually takes place when someone has a limited life expectancy—from less than six months to several years. (Life expectancy must be certified by a doctor.) The patient who pursues a viatical transaction is probably unable to work, and is likely to have a low household income. To reduce money worries, the patient sells the life insurance policy for a lump-sum cash payment—often between 60 to 80 percent of the policy's face value. The payment, which is usually tax-free, goes only to the holder of the policy, who can use the money for any reasons.

The drawbacks of a viatical are that your heirs receive no insurance money, you may not make the best trade available, and the sale is usually not reversible. Before making a decision about your life insurance, think over your options carefully. Talk about this matter with a partner, trusted friend, or a professional financial advisor. For more information, contact the National Viatical Association (see Resources).

BANKRUPTCY

If you try but can't make ends meet, you may have to file bankruptcy. Bankruptcy is a drastic action and a complicated area of the law, so consult a bankruptcy attorney if you're considering it. Legal aid clinics and other non-profit agencies can also provide advice in this area.

Legal Protection in the Workplace

PROTECTING YOUR JOB

You may need to miss work for cancer treatments, follow-up medical visits, and recovery time. You may also need special arrangements to do your job. For these reasons, it is a good idea to let your employer know about your health. When you talk to your supervisor, provide as much information as necessary. That way, everyone involved knows what to expect.

Another strategy is to keep careful records of all talks with your employer or people in the benefits office. List the names of the people you talked with, what you discussed, the date and place you talked, and any conclusions reached. Also, keep copies of your performance reviews. Legal help is available if you feel you have been treated unfairly at work.

People with cancer have the same rights as anyone else in the workplace and should be provided equal opportunities. Hiring, promotion, and treatment in the workplace should depend entirely on ability and qualifications. As long as you are able to fulfill your job duties, you can't be fired for being sick. You also should not have to accept a position you never would have considered before your illness. Most states have laws related to employing people with various illnesses, including some that are specifically aimed at cancer.

AMERICANS WITH DISABILITIES ACT (ADA)

The Americans with Disabilities Act is a federal law enacted in 1990. It protects the rights of people with disabilities. Some people with job problems related to cancer are protected by this act. According to the U.S. Equal Employment Opportunity Commission (EEOC), which administers the ADA, cancer is considered a disability if it is substantially limiting and significantly impairs major life activities.

The ADA prohibits businesses with fifteen or more workers, labor unions, employment agencies, and government agencies from discriminating against someone with a disability who is qualified for a position. The law makes it unlawful to discriminate in employment practices such as recruitment, job application and hiring, training, job assignments, tenure, promotions, pay, benefits, leave, firing, layoff, and all other employment-related activities, terms, conditions, and privileges. The ADA also prohibits screening out disabled employees or the parents of children with disabilities.

Under the ADA, employers are expected to make "reasonable accommodations" that allow disabled persons to do their jobs. A reasonable accommodation is any change or adjustment to a job or work environment that allows a qualified applicant or employee with a disability to participate in the job application process, perform the essential functions of a job, or enjoy the benefits and privileges of employment equal to those enjoyed by employees without disabilities.

Employers are not required to lower standards in order to make accommodations for an employee, nor are they obligated to provide personal use items— such as glasses or hearing aids. However, employers are required to reasonably accommodate qualified applicants or employees with disabilities unless the employer can show it would be an undue hardship to do so. Examples of reasonable accommodations may include:

* Providing or modifying equipment or devices.
* Restructuring a job.
* Offering part-time or modified work schedules.
* Reassigning an employee to a vacant position.

- Adjusting or modifying examinations, training materials, or policies.
- Providing readers and/or interpreters.
- Making the workplace readily accessible to and usable by people with disabilities.

FAMILY AND MEDICAL LEAVE ACT (FMLA)

Under the Family and Medical Leave Act, employers with fifty or more employees must provide up to twelve weeks of unpaid, job-protected leave. The leave can be used to care for yourself or for a family member with a serious illness, including children with cancer. To be covered by the FMLA, you need to tell your employer (and maybe your spouse's employer if you are married) about your health.

Employees are eligible for FMLA protection if they have worked for a covered employer for at least 1,250 hours in the previous twelve months. For the duration of the FMLA leave, the employer must maintain the employee's medical insurance coverage under any company group health plan. If your child has cancer, the pediatric oncologist and the team social worker can help provide needed documentation for your employer.

The FMLA is regulated by the U.S. Department of Labor's Wage and Hour Division, which can provide additional information. Check the telephone directory in your area under U.S. Government, Department of Labor. To file a complaint under this act, contact the U.S. Department of Labor's Employment Standards Administration, Wage and Hour Division. Regional offices are listed in the local telephone book under the Federal Government section.

THE WOMEN'S HEALTH AND CANCER RIGHTS ACT

This 1998 act requires all health plans that cover patients who have undergone mastectomies to also provide breast cancer reconstruction for these patients and to cover prosthetic devices and reconstruction for restoring symmetry. For questions about this new law, contact the U.S. Department of Labor Hotline (see Resources).

WHILE YOU WAIT TO RETURN TO WORK

Perhaps you and your doctor agree that you are not ready to return to work. If you receive funds from a disability plan, read the plan carefully. Find out how long the benefits will last. Also find out if the plan's benefits change over time.

For example, some plans provide benefits for two years if you can't work in your own occupation. Then, after two years they provide benefits only if you can't work in any occupation. If Medicare or Medicaid is covering your health care, it's likely that you will continue to be covered by the same programs.

GETTING INFORMATION

Although a vocational counselor can help with some of your job-related legal questions, you may want to investigate which laws affect you and how you can deal with grievances. To find out more about job accommodations and the employability of people with functional limitations, contact the Job Accommodation Network at 800-526-7234 (http://janweb.icdi.wvu.edu).

If you think you have been discriminated against in employment on the basis of a disability, you can file a complaint with the EEOC within 180 days of the alleged discrimination (according to some state or local laws, you can take up to 300 days). For more specific information about ADA requirements affecting employment, contact the EEOC (see Resources). For general ADA information, answers to specific technical questions, free ADA materials, or information about filing a complaint, contact the Office on the Americans with Disabilities Act (see Resources).

Chapter 10

Cancer Pain in Specific Groups

Mr. Alvarez had colorectal cancer that had spread to his bones. He had fallen and broken a bone in his left arm, but he never asked for pain medicine. His wife knew he must have been in pain. But, when anyone from the health care team asked him about his pain, he replied that he did not need any medicine. When talking to his wife, she explained that Mr. Alvarez came from a family in which the man was the ruler and provider of the house. He did not have time to attend to the children, did not have time for illness, and never showed emotions. She told her husband that she knew he was in pain, but he would not listen to her. This was the way he lived; this was his culture.

Fortunately, there is no longer any need to suffer in silence. No matter what your background or age is, there are many options available for pain relief. Proper pain treatment for people with cancer generally follows established principles and guidelines designed to match pain relief treatments with the severity of pain, while keeping patients as alert, comfortable, and functional as possible. As we have discussed, treatments for pain include a variety of medications, therapies, and nondrug treatments. While these methods are appropriate for treating most cases of cancer pain, some patient populations require special considerations that may alter pain management strategies. These groups include infants and children, the elderly, patients with a history of substance abuse, patients from other cultures, and those with advanced cancer who need palliative care.

Children and Cancer Pain

Although cancer in any person seems like an unfair life event, when the disease strikes a child, the sense of injustice and sadness is heightened. Neither the causes nor the treatment of cancer pain in children are as well studied or as well understood as they are for adults. But, advances in education have greatly improved knowledge about the effectiveness of cancer treatment for children.

Health care professionals and caregivers must not ignore or undertreat pain among younger patients nor underestimate the harmful effects that pain causes. Pain in children should be taken seriously by doctors, nurses, and caregivers and treated aggressively. Yet, too often, children are not provided with adequate pain relief because of mistaken ideas about how they experience and cope with pain. Some health care professionals still incorrectly believe that the nature and causes of cancer-related pain among children are the same as for adults, that identical pain relief strategies apply, or that pain control is less important for children than for adults. Often, since infants and small children cannot express their feelings in adult language, doctors may not interpret emotional expressions as evidence of pain.

At one time, many doctors and other health care professionals accepted the notion that children, especially infants, experience less pain than adults do. Another common misconception among medical professionals has been that children are more susceptible to drug dependence and drug side effects caused by opioid pain medications. Such misconceptions only result in needless suffering among children with cancer. These medications effectively reduce pain regardless of a patient's age, yet rarely cause notable breathing difficulties or result in drug dependence among children. Opioids can even be used safely in very young infants.

Children, regardless of age, feel and suffer from pain. In addition, children do not recover from pain any faster than adults do and they form and remember clear associations between pain and its causes. Just the sight of a needle, for instance, can cause fear, crying, and even panic in anticipation of an injection. Children who know that a doctor's visit is approaching can become upset and tearful hours or even days before the scheduled exam or procedure.

When children struggle with cancer and cancer pain, their situation is aggravated by the sense of helplessness they may feel as they are shuttled to and from

Tests Can Hurt

Most children (about 80 percent) report that they experience pain caused by cancer treatment, and that diagnostic procedures play a large role. Examples of painful diagnostic tests include spinal taps, bone marrow biopsies, and drawing blood for blood tests. These tests and procedures are not only painful, but they must be repeated throughout the cancer treatment experience. This practice exposes children to predictable episodes of pain that they anticipate with dread.

In addition to diagnostic procedures, treatment-related sources of pain for children receiving chemotherapy or radiation include:

- Mouth sores.
- Sore throat.
- Abdominal cramping with diarrhea or constipation.
- Tingling and prickly sensations in hands and feet.
- Muscle cramps.
- Joint pain.

With surgery, there is always acute incisional pain for a few to several days. Infections can also cause pain. Some research suggests that children with cancer pain may be more sensitive to pain from other sources.

unfamiliar environments. Their distress is increased as strangers examine them, question them (if they are old enough to talk), poke and prod them, and often conduct tests or procedures that cause additional pain. Because they have little or no power about decisions regarding their care, children often feel powerless. Also, children may not understand the reasons for tests or procedures. All of these factors fuel children's fear, anxiety, and discomfort. Parents and health care professionals need to take special measures to comfort children before, during, and after tests or treatments, and continually reassure them that their medical care is essential to help them feel better.

Cancer is relatively rare among children, accounting for less than 1 percent of all malignancies. But, many children with cancer suffer cancer-related pain, which can be severe. A child's experience of cancer pain is likely to be very different from that of an adult, primarily because the source of pain usually differs. In adults, pain often develops when solid tumors grow and press on pain sensitive tissue, compress nerves, or block hollow organs. The tumors spread to other parts of the body (metastatic cancer) where they invade other body organs and cause pain. In contrast, solid tumors are much less common in children. Childhood cancers are more commonly *leukemia* (cancers of the blood or blood forming organs) or *lymphoma* (cancer of the lymphatic system). These types of cancer are found in the bloodstream or lymphatic system. They respond quickly to treatment. Only later, if the cancer should recur, does it spread, if at all, to distant organs. This could then result in cancer-related pain.

Anticipating Pain

Painful experiences at the hospital or doctor's office stand out in a child's memory and can lead to anticipatory pain and distress. Anticipatory pain occurs well before a procedure or test is conducted. Since most children are afraid of needles and virtually all of them have received injections, they may become anxious and fearful while waiting for any test or procedure that involves needles. Even when tests cause no physical pain—such as x-rays, CT scans, or MRIs—scheduled procedures may still cause worry and fear. Just the anticipation of returning to the hospital may generate associations with previous painful experiences. Before any visit to the doctor, parents should tell children the reason for the visit and what to expect. All children old enough to talk should be counseled and reassured by caregivers before, during, and after any test or procedure, regardless of whether it causes pain or not. Parents should explain the need for a test or procedure so that the child understands why it is being done and why it is an important part of the medical care plan. Whenever possible, one or both parents should be at their child's side throughout procedures or tests.

Tests and procedures that are insignificant and routine to adults—such as blood draws—can be traumatic for children and create lasting emotional impressions. Parents and health care professionals should not forget that "minor" medical treatment can create tremendous anxiety and fear among children. For relatively common childhood cancers, such as leukemia, diagnostic procedures are painful and may need to be performed frequently. Children with leukemia require spinal taps, during which a needle is inserted into the spine to remove spinal fluid (see Chapter 2). Routine blood tests that cause little concern for most adults take on far greater significance for children, who associate needles with pain. Fear and anxiety may translate into less cooperation and multiple attempts may be needed, which only increases a child's aversion to medical procedures.

REACTIONS TO PAIN IN CHILDREN

Parents of children who are in pain may feel fearful, helpless, or angry. They may believe that increased pain signals a worsening of their child's cancer, although pain intensity and severity of cancer are not necessarily related. In fact, significant pain may result after successful cancer treatment. Parents may downplay the severity of a child's pain in an attempt to help the child cope with the seriousness of the illness. But, children can sense when a parent becomes anxious and upset about their illness and treatment. Such perceptions may cause children—even very young ones—to hide or deny their pain and not admit they hurt in an attempt to protect their parents' feelings. Children who have previously been ill may worry that pain indicates a progression of disease, or they might associate the expression of pain with subsequent medical tests, causing them to understate pain levels to avoid painful procedures.

For some families, pain may actually become the focus of attention, which can lead to even greater anxiety and possible depression. Anxious and depressed patients, whether children or adults, are likely to experience greater pain.

A child's perception of pain is also greatly affected by social factors, such as family support and stability, and financial stresses placed on families by cancer treatment. Children may feel guilty if they perceive that they are the source of family problems or if they believe they are to blame for their own pain (i.e., their own misbehavior or mischievous thoughts caused the disease). Using age-appropriate terms to explain why children are having pain is therefore important, even when children are quite young.

PAIN ASSESSMENT IN CHILDREN

The criteria for evaluating children's pain are similar to those used for adults. Initial pain assessments typically consist of a comprehensive history and physical examination, including questions about the type, location, and severity of pain and the steps parents have taken to control it. Yet, evaluating children often presents unique challenges, especially if patients are too young to communicate verbally.

The capacity of children to communicate varies considerably. As they grow, their ability to verbally communicate information about their pain increases. By the age of six, many children can describe pain severity, location, duration, and type. Some may be evaluated with the same visual analog scales used with adults (see Chapter 3).

There are also pain scales used specifically for children. For example, the "Oucher" scale shows a measure from 0 to 100 and six photographs of a four-year-old's face displaying different expressions, each corresponding to a different level of pain intensity. Other child-oriented pain scales match different colors to pain intensity or use poker chips to represent "pieces of hurt." The evaluator asks children how many chips their pain has. For teenagers, a list of words describing types of pain may be useful.

Some children are quite capable of telling doctors, nurses, and caregivers where and how much they hurt. Some can describe various characteristics of their pain, discriminate among different types of pain sensations, report how their pain changes throughout the day, and link specific activities that cause increased or decreased pain. Others have great difficulty talking about their sensations. Pain behaviors also change as children develop. For example, an infant may respond to pain with generalized movements, changes in facial expressions, and crying, whereas toddlers can signal the location of their pain, and older children are generally capable of describing their pain in some detail, or at least indicating pain severity from a rating scale.

Infants and very young children cannot communicate the location or intensity of their pain, which makes pain assessment particularly challenging. The only way infants express pain is to cry, but this behavior may also signal hunger or a wet diaper rather than pain. Doctors often must judge pain intensity from a child's behavior and from physiological signs, such as breathing rate, heart rate, and palm sweating, as well as from parents' reports. Parents should carefully observe a child, paying particular attention to facial expressions, unusual behavior, and any other signs that may indicate pain.

Even when parents watch a young child, they may find it difficult to gauge pain level. Some children, even those capable of talking, may not complain or cry, which makes pain assessment even more difficult. Silence in the presence of pain may indicate that a child has given up hope and requires emotional support from caregivers and medical personnel. Parents and health care professionals must keep watch for other signs of pain, discomfort, or distress. Older children may cry not just as a result of pain, but also because they are afraid or anxious about upcoming tests or procedures. For doctors, nurses, and caregivers, making the distinction can be difficult. In either case, a child in distress requires attention. *When children appear to be in pain, they should be treated as if they are, even when parents or doctors are unsure.*

MANAGING CANCER PAIN IN CHILDREN

Procedural Pain

For children with cancer, procedures and tests are the worst part of having the disease because they cause a great deal of pain and are repeated regularly. Children vividly remember the pain caused by a procedure and anticipate the prospect of returning for another one with dread. In these situations, the pain is acute, not chronic. The anxiety and fear brought on by such procedures does not decrease over time. Procedural pain is a real and frightening problem for children, but many health care professionals do not take it seriously enough. As a result, many young patients suffer needlessly.

Acute pain caused by procedures and tests can be minimized using a combination of drug therapy, nondrug pain relief techniques, and lots of reassurance from parents and the medical staff. For example, a child undergoing a spinal tap to collect spinal fluid may benefit from a detailed explanation of what to expect, a local anesthetic cream over the puncture site, relaxation and distraction, an antianxiety medicine, and a strong, short-acting analgesic. Some health care professionals advise parents to discuss the procedure with their child afterwards to build trust and further explain why their treatment is so important. The choices of pain treatments vary, depending on the amount of pain expected during a procedure as well as on an individual child's level of anxiety or fear. For more invasive procedures, such as bone marrow sampling, a general anesthetic may be necessary to make the child unconscious during the test.

Another pain control technique specially designed for children is conscious sedation in which just enough medication is given (preferably by mouth) to decrease pain caused by procedures or tests. But, it allows children to remain conscious enough to respond to voice commands and questions.

Drug Therapy

Principles of pain control for children are similar to those applied to adults. Chronic pain caused by cancer can usually be controlled with oral pain medications, including acetaminophen, NSAIDs, and opioid analgesics. Most analgesic medications used for adults work well in children (at lower doses). Two NSAIDs, tolmetin and naproxen, are specifically approved by the U.S. Food and Drug Administration for treating children. NSAIDs are particularly effective for treating mild to moderate pain caused by inflammation or bone tumors. However, these medications should not be prescribed for children who are at risk for internal bleeding. Children should not receive aspirin because it increases the risk of Reyes Syndrome, a potentially serious and life-threatening condition. Your doctor will tell you if your child is old enough to take aspirin.

Just as with adult patients, opioids are the mainstay of treatment for moderate to severe pain. Doctors may also prescribe antidepressants, stimulants, and corticosteroids to enhance pain relief. Pain medications for children should be administered on a strict schedule around the clock, not just as needed, to ensure that sufficient levels of analgesics remain in the bloodstream throughout the day. Ideally, pain medications are given orally to avoid pain caused by needle sticks. (Some medicines can be crushed and placed in food or drinks.) Young children cannot connect the pain of injection with future relief, and many would rather live with their pain than get injections. When injections are necessary, doctors or nurses can apply an anesthetic cream over the injection site to minimize pain. If children refuse to take medicines by mouth, alternatives include opioid patches, suppositories and—as a last resort—intravenous or intramuscular injections. Refusal to take medications orally may mean that children are exercising the last bit of control they have during a process about which they feel helpless.

Doctors rarely use nerve blocks or surgical procedures to relieve a child's pain. But, when necessary, these techniques work well. In fact, nerve blocks and morphine given into the epidural space of the spine have been used successfully in very young babies. Some pain control options that are suitable for adults are inappropriate for children. For example, regional anesthesia is not a reasonable solution for most children because their pain often occurs across a large area of the body and is hard to pinpoint.

As with adults, the risk of drug dependence or addiction among children is extremely low and should not prevent doctors from prescribing opioids. Some doctors still mistakenly believe that opioids should not be prescribed to young children. In most cases, weak and strong opioids can be combined with other medications to produce adequate pain relief. Some types of constant pain are managed better by continued opioid infusion, even for children who are at home. This method of drug delivery requires a doctor to surgically place a catheter just under the skin and into a large vein (see Chapter 4). A special pump attached to the catheter dispenses medications automatically at regular intervals. The technique eliminates the need for repeated injections. Children as young as five have been taught to use patient-controlled analgesia. They decide when intravenous medications are needed and they push a button to cause the medicine to flow through the catheter into their bloodstream.

Nondrug Techniques of Pain Relief

Many of the same nondrug pain relief methods that have proven to be effective for adults can be altered appropriately to provide relief for children (see Chapter 7). Such techniques include biofeedback, relaxation therapy, distraction, desensitization, hypnosis, and psychological counseling for both patients and families. Children are particularly responsive to distraction because it involves imagination and "pretending." Children also respond well to music and being rocked, massaged, or stroked during painful periods. Applying heat or cold to sensitive areas can also be effective. Although nondrug techniques cannot eliminate pain completely, they often reduce pain to some extent and may enhance the effects of medication.

Reassurance and Support

Reassuring and comforting children before their very first cancer-related procedure is an effective strategy to help reduce anxiety and fear before and during future procedures. One or both parents should be present before, during, and after treatment to offer reassurance and help the child calm down and relax. Research shows that children having procedures greatly benefit from having a parent present to provide a sense of security and lessen fears of abandonment.

Reducing Anxiety About the Treatment Setting

When a child is diagnosed and treated for cancer, both the patient and family enter the complex and often frightening world of modern medicine. Hospitals and major medical centers can be vast and confusing places with seemingly endless corridors and multiple buildings. Hospital rooms can be drab and scary. Many professionals have questions to ask, tests to perform, and treatments to give. A heightened sense of anxiety can intensify a child's perception of pain.

With time and experience, however, parents and children become familiar with the medical centers and other places where treatment is given. They memorize the route and all the shortcuts from home to the hospital. They master the way to the cafeteria. They find the spots that offer privacy. They bring blankets and pictures from home to brighten rooms. They learn to pack snacks and toys and books for clinic visits. They learn to navigate the miles of hallways. The staff become real people and some important relationships are formed. Children with cancer and their parents adjust to their new world and learn what to expect.

Explaining routines, tests, procedures, and treatment can help reduce children's fears about what is happening to them. The following are suggestions to help patients and families understand and adjust to the health care system:

- Ask for maps or a tour of the hospital.
- Have professionals explain the part they play in providing care.
- Determine exactly where treatment will take place.
- Make hospital rooms as homey as possible.
- Have activities on hand for time spent in clinic.
- Clarify the role of the child's referring doctor.
- Check on insurance or managed care requirements.
- Request definitions of unfamiliar terms.
- Review the written materials provided by the team.
- Ask team members to describe how the "system" works.
- Talk to other children and parents to see what worked for them.

Children should not be left alone in treatment or hospital rooms for long periods so they don't dwell on their worries, their pain, or scheduled procedures.

Parents should remain calm during tests and procedures, since children take their cues from adults. A parent who appears nervous or fearful will have a far more difficult time settling down a child than one who appears relaxed and confident. Often, simply offering factual information about a procedure is an effective strategy because it returns some sense of control and realistic expectations to a child. Having a greater sense of control can reduce some of the feelings of helplessness associated with having cancer and undergoing painful procedures. Distractions such as books or toys may also be useful to lower anxiety and pass the time while waiting for a procedure. If the child is old enough to understand, parents should explain in detail what to expect during the upcoming treatment. A child's fantasies are often worse than reality.

During diagnostic and therapeutic procedures, children should have adequate privacy. Health care professionals should ensure that they feel comfortable and secure. Parents can help by bringing familiar items from home, such as favorite toys, pictures, books, or stuffed animals. Music, video games, and television are also effective distractions for children. For hospitalized children, the health care team and parents may want to schedule "safe times" during which the child can rest assured that no procedures or tests will be performed.

Cancer Pain in the Elderly

Older people who have cancer deserve thorough and aggressive pain management. Yet, misconceptions and inappropriate beliefs about how this group experiences and copes with pain often impede appropriate care. According to pain control guidelines issued by the government, the elderly are at-risk for the undertreatment of cancer pain.

Many people assume that increased pain is a normal part of the aging process—a condition to be endured without complaint. Some health care professionals wrongly believe that older people are less sensitive to pain and that they cannot tolerate opioid pain medications well. While it is true that older adults are likely to experience more chronic pain than younger ones, particularly in the muscles and joints, there is no reason to ignore pain or leave it untreated.

Pain is extremely common among older people, and it often goes undetected. An estimated 25 to 50 percent of elderly people have chronic pain problems. For nursing home residents, it is estimated that 45 to 80 percent have substantial pain that is untreated. This group often requires special considerations with regard to pain assessment and treatment because of physiological and psychological changes that occur with aging. While many elderly people experience pain, there is no reason to ignore it or consider it any less serious simply because of a patient's age. Health care professionals should pursue pain management aggressively for elderly patients. Caregivers or people with cancer who feel that their reports of pain do not result in adequate attention should speak frankly with a doctor or nurse on the health care team.

PAIN ASSESSMENT IN ELDERLY PATIENTS

Accurately assessing pain among elderly patients poses some unique challenges. Older people tend to understate the amount of pain they experience and may need to be prompted several times before they provide an accurate description of the severity and type of their pain. Some older patients are reluctant to complain about pain or to display behaviors that indicate they are in pain. This may occur because older individuals often live with one or more conditions that cause pain, such as arthritis, so they do not pay particular attention to new pain, considering it yet another burden of aging they must endure. This attitude also makes assessment of pain related specifically to cancer more difficult for health professionals, because patients may wait until pain becomes too severe before they visit a doctor.

Some degree of mental impairment is present in an estimated 5 percent of patients sixty-five years and older, and in more than 20 percent of those older than eighty years. Patients with mental impairment, such as Alzheimer's disease, may be unable to discuss their pain or provide adequate information to doctors or nurses. They may not remember when their pain starts, how severe it becomes, or what measures bring relief. Their reports of pain may change often and quickly. As a result, elderly patients often require pain assessments more frequently than younger ones. Patients with diminished mental functioning or who have difficulty verbalizing thoughts may be better able to describe their pain through the use of simplified pain scales (see Chapter 3).

Older patients may have hearing and vision difficulties, making communication with caregivers and medical personnel more difficult. And the pain and pain treatment may also contribute to the inability of elderly patients to accurately describe their condition. Opioids often dull a person's mental ability and decrease alertness, as can the presence of pain itself.

Doctors and nurses can learn important information by assessing pain before and after a patient receives analgesics to determine the effectiveness of treatment. But for elderly patients who do not communicate well, doctors might have to rely on caregivers to observe behavioral changes that signal whether pain has decreased, remained constant, or increased after therapy.

MANAGING CANCER PAIN IN THE ELDERLY

Strategies for managing pain in elderly people with cancer follow the same fundamental principles used for treating younger adults. Yet, misconceptions about pain in older patients often lead to inadequate treatment. For instance, elderly patients in pain are frequently given only nonopioid medications or weak doses of opioids instead of strong ones because their health care professionals mistakenly believe they cannot tolerate the effects of more potent opioids. Or, they may discount an older patient's complaints of pain because of the widespread notion that pain is a natural and expected consequence of aging.

The cornerstone of treatment for cancer pain among elderly patients is drug therapy, just as it is for younger patients. Acetaminophen, aspirin, NSAIDs, and opioids should be administered in doses that match the severity and type of pain, as outlined in the *Three-Step Analgesic Ladder for Cancer Pain Management* (see Chapter 4). Treatment may be supplemented with adjuvant medications, such as antianxiety medications, antidepressants, and steroids. But some important considerations must be kept in mind when treating elderly patients with medications.

Most pain medications are metabolized (processed) by the liver and kidneys. In elderly people, these and other organs tend to function less efficiently and are more dramatically affected by medications. In addition, the elderly generally have less water and muscle mass and more body fat than younger adults. These differences mean that older patients may not tolerate doses of analgesics as well as younger ones. So, determining the most effective dose can be a challenge for doctors. NSAIDs may cause more side effects among elderly patients, including high blood pressure, kidney problems, dizziness, confusion, and excessive salt and water retention. Elderly patients who begin taking NSAIDs should be watched closely for good kidney function.

An advantage to lower drug tolerance among the elderly is that lower doses often achieve adequate pain relief and last longer. "Rescue" doses of opioids to control breakthrough pain may be lower among elderly patients. Doctors usually begin pain medications at lower doses for elderly people with cancer and increase them more gradually than they would for younger patients. This precaution not only decreases the chances for drug-related side effects, but also lessens the risk of adverse reactions caused by mixing pain medicines with other medicines patients may already be taking.

Some doctors still believe that elderly patients shouldn't receive opioids or they will only prescribe them at very low doses. The result is often inadequate pain relief. While it is true that older people are more sensitive to the effects of opioids, these medications should still play a very important role in cancer pain relief, regardless of a patient's age. Elderly patients are likely to experience grogginess and sedation when opioid treatment begins, however, these side effects usually diminish shortly after the start of drug therapy. Mild respiratory depression (shallow breathing) may also occur, but this is no reason to discontinue opioid therapy.

Opioids may also cause nausea and vomiting, which can be relieved with appropriate antiemetic (antinausea) medications. To reduce constipation associated

Family Members Can Help

Family members are often crucial to successful pain management among elderly patients.

Caregivers, who may be elderly themselves, often assume significant burdens when caring for an elderly cancer patient. They must be sure that the patient takes the correct pain medicine on time and at the prescribed dose, monitor the patient for changes in pain status (such as the emergence of breakthrough pain), and keep in touch with members of the health care team. This can be a demanding and exhausting responsibility. Some caregivers may require the assistance of home nursing, home hospice services, home health aides, and volunteers (see Resources) to assume some of their duties, provide periodic rests, and ease their physical and psychological stress.

with opioids, doctors usually prescribe laxatives as soon as a patient begins taking opioids (see Chapter 6). Because older individuals are usually less physically active, drink less fluid than younger ones, and are more likely to take other medications that cause constipation, laxatives are particularly important to keep patients comfortable.

Alternate routes of drug delivery are available for elderly patients who cannot take medications orally, including suppositories and intravenous administration. Chemical and surgical nerve blocks are just as effective in elderly patients as they are in younger ones, but older patients may not tolerate the side effects of these procedures very well and may require longer recovery periods. Patient-controlled analgesia is useful for some elderly patients but should be closely monitored by the health care team or caregivers at home.

Elderly patients often take multiple medications to treat other conditions in addition to cancer. As more medications are added to the list, the risk of adverse and potentially dangerous drug interactions increases. To minimize the threat, patients must inform doctors of all the medications they are taking, including any vitamins or herbal preparations.

Elderly patients or their caregivers should maintain regular and frequent contact with members of the health care team to closely monitor drug effectiveness and drug-related side effects, and to make changes to the program as needed. Reassessment of pain management programs should be done whenever elderly patients move to a new setting, such as from the hospital to home, or when changes to the pain therapy program are made.

EMOTIONAL AND PSYCHOLOGICAL ISSUES OF PAIN IN THE ELDERLY

Elderly patients require a significant amount of emotional support to deal with cancer and its treatment. If symptoms of cancer, including pain, are not addressed, older patients are more likely than others to suffer chronic pain, depression, sleep disturbances, impaired ability to walk, falls, slow rehabilitation, problems caused by taking multiple medications, mental impairment, and malnutrition.

A high number of patients who suffer chronic pain also experience depression and anxiety at some time during cancer treatment. Doctors should consider these factors when planning a pain relief program for elderly patients. As discussed earlier, depression often causes patients to experience greater pain (see Chapter 9). Doctors and other members of the health care team should recognize the source of pain and pursue pain relief aggressively, taking into account the emotional state of a patient.

A carefully designed pain relief program will consider all of the current knowledge about pain relieving medications and other treatments as well as the physical and psychological effects that may result from their use. When properly planned and carried out, pain therapy for the elderly can greatly reduce and even eliminate pain and discomfort, which frees them to pursue daily activities and greatly improve the quality of their life.

Treatment Issues for People with a History of Substance Abuse

Cancer patients who have a history of alcohol or drug abuse require special attention when they undergo drug therapy to relieve pain. Patients are responsible for being honest and informing their doctors, other members of the health care team, and caregivers if they have any history (current or past) of substance abuse. Patients serve their own best interests by being candid with their health care team. If they hold back information about their current or past drug abuse, patients risk getting medication doses that are too low to relieve pain. To be assured that they receive adequate pain control therapy, patients should discuss these issues with a doctor or nurse.

Some doctors are reluctant to prescribe opioids to patients who abuse or have abused drugs in the past, fearing that the patient will become addicted. The result can be undertreatment of pain. As discussed earlier, the risk of addiction from cancer pain medication in the general population is extremely low, affecting less than 1 percent of patients who have no history of substance abuse (see Chapter 4). The risk increases substantially among those who have abused drugs or alcohol. However, this is no reason to withhold medications, even strong opioids such as morphine, from cancer patients in pain. Doctors must weigh the pain relieving benefits of drug therapy against the risks of dependence for each patient.

One strategy to reduce the chances of developing a drug habit again is for the doctor to first rely on medications such as NSAIDs and steroids for mild to moderate pain, which are not habit forming. Most importantly, patients must communicate frequently with their health care team to let them know about the effectiveness of pain relief measures. If stronger medications are needed to control pain, doctors should be willing to prescribe them, regardless of whether a patient has a history of substance abuse. However, doctors should insist that drugs be taken precisely as prescribed—meaning on time and at the correct dosage. Doctors may also ask patients to keep pain medication diaries to demonstrate their ability to adhere to the drug therapy plan. Caregivers can play an important role by supervising the administration of opioids to prevent abuse.

Doctors may not trust pain intensity reports by cancer patients who are at risk for drug abuse, suspecting that they may exaggerate their reports of pain severity in order to get higher doses of opioids. However, health professionals with a great deal of experience treating people in pain have reported that though a small number of patients lie about pain levels so that they can get higher drug doses, most take medicines reliably and in correct amounts.

Patients who use their pain medications improperly or make awkward excuses about why their prescriptions run low ahead of schedule risk losing their doctors' trust and may not receive adequate pain control in the future. If drugs are used as prescribed, there should be no need for early refills. Another strategy doctors may choose is to prescribe only a week's worth of pain medication at a time to reduce the chances that patients will take extra opioids.

Doctors may prefer to prescribe long-acting opioids to be taken on a regular schedule rather than prescribing short-acting medications "as needed." Longer-acting opioids provide more consistent pain relief and tend not to produce "highs" associated with the shorter-acting medications. Patients who are recovered addicts may worry about starting therapy with medications that can potentially lead to dependence. These individuals require reassurance and close supervision during drug therapy.

Cancer patients with a history of substance abuse may require help from medical professionals who are knowledgeable about both cancer pain and drug dependence. Doctors may instruct patients who are at home to work with psychiatric and substance abuse counselors to ensure that they stick to prescribed drug therapy and prevent drug abuse. Substance abusers, more than patients in other groups, may also require psychological counseling for mental health problems.

Culturally Diverse Groups

Cultural background has a powerful influence on how people react to and cope with pain and illness. It often affects how patients express and rate pain, what significance pain has, how acceptable it is to have others present during doctor visits, how a person normally copes with pain, and what traditional or folk remedies a patient uses or has used in the past. For instance, in some cultures, the vocal expression of pain is considered weak behavior. For those who have such beliefs, enduring pain may be considered a sign of strength. Men, in particular, may be expected to endure pain and discomfort without complaining. It cannot be assumed that people who don't talk about pain aren't suffering or won't benefit from pain therapy.

People in other cultural groups may be more vocal about their pain and think nothing of displaying their discomfort as a way to bring relief, and they may even demand pain control. Expressions of crying and moaning can be ways of attempting to relieve pain and may not accurately reflect the severity of distress. In some cultural traditions, people believe that pain is the result of supernatural powers, fate, punishment for previous deeds, evil spirits, or witchcraft, and that it is closely associated with death. To some patients, the pain may be as significant as the illness itself.

To provide the best care, health professionals must consider their patients' cultural backgrounds and how they might affect pain assessment and pain treatment. Unfortunately, the U.S. health care system generally lacks sensitivity to various cultural or religious differences that may affect how patients express pain and how pain fits into patients' world views. The result can be poor communication, inadequate treatment, and increased pain and suffering. Pain relief strategies that incorporate an individual's cultural beliefs about pain have a much better chance of success.

IMPACT ON CARE

Cultural influences significantly affect communication between patient and provider and impact the success of pain management plans. For instance, a patient who comes from a culture in which pain endurance is associated with strength and character may not be easily convinced to take prescribed pain medications. Health care providers who are aware of and who adjust to cultural differences

Pain Control in Minority Populations

According to the federal government (Agency for Healthcare Research and Quality), in general, minority patients are likely to receive less adequate treatment for cancer pain than nonminorities. Research has shown that African Americans and Hispanics with pain due to metastatic cancer were three times more likely to receive inadequate pain treatment than nonminorities.

The barriers that impede pain control among minority groups may include:

- Cultural differences.
- Language differences, causing health professionals to judge pain levels based on behavior rather than on a patient's description (often resulting in underestimation of pain).
- Inaccurate and incomplete pain assessment.
- Less frequent follow-up care by medical professionals.
- Decreased access to appropriate medical care.
- Fear of addiction to opioid pain medications among patients.
- Reluctance of doctors to prescribe opioid pain medications.
- Economic disadvantages among minority populations.
- Inadequate insurance reimbursement for pain treatment.

among their patients are in a position to provide the most effective care to patients who are in pain.

Research indicates that minority patients are less likely than those from nonminority groups to receive the pain treatment they need. According to the World Health Organization, for instance, African Americans and Hispanics with pain caused by metastatic cancer (cancer that has spread to different parts of the body) were three times more likely to receive inadequate pain treatment than were nonminority patients. Other researchers have also found that patients' ethnic backgrounds affect their level of pain management. One study found that African Americans and Hispanic people with cancer were likely to receive inadequate pain treatment compared with whites. They reported that doctors underestimated the severity of pain for 64 percent of the Hispanic patients and 74 percent of the African-American patients, and they were also more likely to underestimate the severity of pain for female patients than for male patients.[1]

The differences may be related to socioeconomic status, education, access to health care, knowledge, attitudes toward doctors, patient behavior, and other factors. Cultural and language differences may also play a role because they can inhibit communication and understanding between patients and doctors (see Chapter 1). The result may be inadequate pain assessment, pain treatment, and follow-up care.

Because people from minority cultures may behave differently in the presence of pain (such as not complaining), health care providers may misjudge a patient's level of distress and therefore not treat pain aggressively. Cultural influences among minority groups may also cause patients to wait longer to seek out treatment for pain or to first visit traditional folk healers before seeing a doctor who practices western medical techniques.

Some health care professionals may be more concerned about the potential for drug addiction in minority patients who require opioids to control pain, although there is no evidence to suggest that minority groups are more likely to misuse pain relief drugs. Some researchers have even observed that minority patients, particularly those who are African American or Hispanic, have substantial difficulty obtaining commonly prescribed pain relief drugs from the neighborhood pharmacies in low-income neighborhoods, which often carry limited supplies of opioids because of the threat of robbery.[2]

Cultural sensitivity is growing within the medical community as health care professionals become more aware of the importance of culture. But, patients should not assume that their health care professionals are familiar with personal and cultural factors that have an impact on how they experience and cope with pain. People with cancer or their caregivers whose cultures differ from those in the United States should speak with members of their health care team so that

---

[1] K. O. Anderson, T. R. Mendoza, V. Valero, S. P. Richman, C. Russell, J. Hurley, C. DeLeon, P. Washington, G. Palos, R. Payne, and C. S. Cleeland, "Minority cancer patients and their providers: pain management attitudes and practice," *Cancer*, 88 (2000): 1929–1938.

[2] R. S. Morrison, S. Wallenstein, D. K. Natale, R. S. Senzel, and L. Huang, "We don't carry that"— Failures of pharmacies in predominantly nonwhite neighborhoods to stock opioid analgesics," *New England J Medicine*, 342 (2000): 1023–1026.

doctors are aware of factors that might affect pain assessment and treatment decisions. You will benefit if you discuss your own personal way of dealing with pain and how your cultural background may influence your behavior.

Ideally, all members of your oncology team should be nonjudgmental, flexible, sensitive, and respectful of any cultural differences you may have and should identify your health-related cultural beliefs and practices. To bridge cultural gaps, you should discuss your needs and wishes to ensure that you receive the best and most comprehensive care possible. With this knowledge, your doctor can develop a pain management plan that takes into account needs based on your cultural background. Staying silent about your beliefs can jeopardize the success of your treatment and can result in unnecessary pain and suffering.

Palliative Care

"I still remember the day I received the call from Tom, my fifty-year-old brother, telling me he had a recurrence of melanoma. His disease had already spread to both lungs. We had many long talks in the days that followed. We spoke about the possibility of his death and he told me that his biggest fear was dying in pain. I reassured him that everything possible would be done to control his pain. He was more than my brother, he was a best friend."

Susan, a cancer nurse

Palliative care is treatment that provides support and relieves symptoms, but is not expected to cure the disease. The main purpose is to improve the patient's quality of life. It is traditionally an option for critically ill individuals whose disease is considered incurable and are nearing the end of life. Palliative care may be provided in varied environments, including hospices, community-based palliative care units, designated beds within hospitals, and even a patient's home. The goal of palliative care for cancer patients is comfort and pain relief, not a cure.

Patients with a life-threatening disease such as cancer may have difficulty shifting from traditional care to palliative care, knowing that their health care team can no longer cure their disease. Family members and other caregivers may feel guilty about the transition. Regarding palliative care, the World Health Organization reported that "Control of pain, of other symptoms, and of psychological, social and spiritual problems, is paramount. The goal of palliative care is achievement of the best quality of life for patients and their families. Many aspects of palliative care are also applicable earlier in the course of the illness in conjunction with anticancer treatment."[3]

Palliative care should include not only medical treatments to relieve pain, but also emotional support for patients and their loved ones. Psychologists and counselors can provide both preparatory grief counseling and bereavement counseling in the case of a patient who is terminally ill. Issues of loss that are present during advanced disease should be discussed with a mental health professional beginning early in the course of treatment and throughout the course of the illness.

Many patients do not receive adequate pain management even at the end of life. Relieving pain among this group should be of the highest priority for health professionals and caregivers, because pain relief greatly improves the quality of one's life regardless of how serious the illness. An estimated 70 to 90 percent of persons with advanced cancer experience pain—pain that can be eliminated or at least reduced. Yet in many cases, and for a variety of reasons, some doctors are still reluctant to use all of the tools at their disposal to treat pain.

Patients and caregivers should insist on adequate pain relief. One of the barriers to adequate pain relief, is fear of dependence on opioid medications (see Chapter 1). Yet among patients with advanced cancer, this concern should have no influence on the decision to prescribe opioids, even at very high doses, if they bring comfort.

HOSPICE CARE

"The day came when Tom's melanoma spread to his central nervous system and his pain escalated dramatically. He was admitted to a hospital near my home and the "nightmare" began. My first indication of a problem came with a call from Tom at 4:00 AM one morning. As I answered the phone, I heard him say, "the pain is unbearable and they say there isn't anything else that can be done." I dressed and went to the hospital and from that day until his death, my sister and I took turns staying at his side. We served as his advocates in his struggle for pain relief that followed."

[3] *Cancer Pain Relief.* Geneva: World Health Organization, 1996.

Finding Hospice Care

Ask a doctor, nurse, or social worker to give you a list of local hospices. Hospice services are also listed in the yellow pages of the telephone book. There are agencies that can refer you to hospices in your community, such as the American Cancer Society, the Hospice Foundation of America, the National Association for Home Care, and the National Hospice and Palliative Care Organization. See the Resources section at the end of this book for contact information.

Hospice is a philosophy of care for terminally ill patients in which health care providers and caregivers strive to keep patients pain free, alert, and as comfortable as possible. Hospice care is appropriate when a person with cancer can no longer benefit from attempts to cure the disease. The patient, family, and doctor can decide together when to begin hospice services. If the illness improves or goes into remission, a patient can leave hospice care and resume curative treatments. Hospice care can resume at any time. Hospice care is not necessarily conducted at a specific location. Care can take place in a number of settings, including a patient's home, a hospital, a nursing home, or a private hospice facility.

Hospice is a concept whose origins can be traced hundreds of years back to the idea of offering a place of shelter and rest to weary and sick travelers on a long journey—a place of hospitality. In 1967, the term was first applied to the care of dying patients. Hospice care focuses on providing humane and compassionate care for people in the last phases of an incurable disease so that they may live as fully and comfortably as possible surrounded by loved ones. It is appropriate when the patient can no longer benefit from attempts to cure cancer. Hospice care centers on treating the person, not the disease, and emphasizes quality rather than length of life.

Typically, hospice care involves an interdisciplinary health care team of doctors, nurses, social workers, counselors, hospice-certified nursing assistants, clergy, therapists, and volunteers—each offering support based on their own area of expertise. Together, they provide comprehensive palliative care aimed at relieving symptoms, controlling pain, and providing supportive social, emotional, and spiritual care services.

"The first hurdle with Tom's oncologist was overcome and he was started on a morphine drip with instructions that it be increased as needed. The next obstacle was with several members of the nursing staff. As a nurse, myself, this was a huge disappointment to me. Entire eight-hour shifts passed with my sister and I asking for the dose to be increased without success. One nurse actually asked me if I was "trying to kill" my brother. His agony resulted not only from his untreated pain, but was intensified when the staff appeared not to believe his reports of pain. He was alert and expressed his feelings, but to little avail."

Terminally ill patients may experience severe pain or other symptoms, including profound psychological distress. In some cases, symptom management requires high doses of opioids and other types of pain relief medications. The goal of pain management for patients whose disease is advanced and who are in severe pain, is to increase comfort while allowing them to remain in control of their life. This means that side effects are managed to ensure that patients experience as little pain as possible, yet remain alert enough to make decisions that they feel are important. However, high doses of opioids often result in a trade-off between adequate pain control and decreased alertness, functional ability, and side effects of medication, such as confusion and hallucinations.

Sometimes, however, adequate pain management cannot be achieved without decreasing a patient's alertness. For example, high doses of opioids and sedatives may be needed to control pain. Side effects such as continual drowsiness and prolonged periods of sleep may be unavoidable in such cases. Any pain symptom that a patient finds intolerable should be taken very seriously and addressed aggressively with appropriate pain management techniques. If the patient's regular doctor cannot find a solution, caregivers may decide to consult with a pain management expert to find solutions.

If severe pain persists after doctors have explored all potential alternatives, the patient and family may consider terminal sedation in order to relieve suffering. The patient may have specified his or her desires on this matter in an advance directive, which may include detailed terms of care (see Chapter 11). The main objective of terminal sedation is to preserve a patient's comfort, which may require that the patient be asleep most of the day. A secondary, unplanned effect of this may be hastening the end of life because continuous sedation can impair the functioning of the heart and lungs.

Terminal sedation is different from euthanasia, which is illegal in the United States. Aggressive steps to relieve pain, including terminal sedation, are sometimes appropriate. Terminal sedation is legally recognized and ethically justified in the care of the terminally ill. Psychological counseling with mental health professionals may aid loved ones under these difficult circumstances. If family members disagree on whether to take measures that could hasten the death of a patient yet will greatly ease pain, they should consider, whenever possible, the patient's preferences.

Terminal sedation can involve one of several pharmacologic options. If the patient is currently being treated with opioids, the opioid dose will usually be increased as a first step. But tolerance to opioids and severe pain can rule out this option. Sometimes a side effect of increasing the opioid dose may occur as well, such as severe muscle twitching. In these cases an adjuvant analgesic such as a neuroleptic, benzodiazepine, or barbiturate may be added.

"From the beginning of his illness, taking control of the situation was very important to Tom. He took great satisfaction in making informed decisions and always having a plan. His plan was rewritten many, many times, and each new plan had fresh hope. His final plan was for a peaceful, pain-free death with dignity. However, the presence of unrelieved pain took away his control and any remaining independence. That made me very sad. The end was painful and emotionally upsetting for my sister and I. Tom suffered silently, mourning the pain and the indignity. For him, I'm glad he's at peace; but he needn't have had to suffer the way he did."

CHAPTER 11

Regulatory, Legislative, and Ethical Issues:

EFFECTS ON PEOPLE WITH CANCER PAIN

"When you are in this circumstance [dealing with cancer], you know for the most part that your friends and family will continue to love you, but it's the strangers who show you love that gives you faith in mankind. It makes you feel like maybe you can beat this."
Alberta, a cancer survivor

Cancer is just as much a political issue, as it is a medical, social, psychological, and economic one. Policy makers at all levels of government make decisions that have the potential to impact the lives of over eight million Americans that now have cancer or a history of cancer.

The American Cancer Society (ACS) has traditionally been a vigorous advocate for people with cancer and their families in national and state efforts to formulate public policy. A range of legislative efforts are currently underway in Congress and various state houses that have the potential to significantly affect the ways in which the public, providers, and health systems understand the issue of cancer pain control, and obtain and use appropriate and adequate cancer pain treatment. Among the legislative issues currently being addressed are coverage, adequate reimbursement for pain control, access to pain specialists, and support for health professional education about and adoption of nationwide guidelines by the Agency for Healthcare Research and Quality (AHRQ).

Continued action on several legislative fronts is necessary if real progress is to be made. Support for legislation for pain control medication reimbursement by private payers and Medicare/Medicaid will help to ensure access to pain treatment by all Americans. Advocacy for additional research funding for agencies that conduct cancer pain research will ensure that knowledge and understanding of pain control issues will continue to improve. Clear positions are needed on public policy issues that affect the public's willingness to ask for and obtain adequate pain treatment.

Oregon Death with Dignity Act

At the state level, legislation has been passed that has affected the quality of pain management. In 1994, residents of the state of Oregon voted narrowly to approve the Death with Dignity Act. The law currently allows doctors to actively and intentionally assist terminally ill patients with ending their lives. Under the Act, a competent adult citizen of the state of Oregon who has a terminal illness that is expected to cause death within six months may obtain and self-administer a lethal dose of drugs prescribed by a doctor specifically for the purpose of ending the patient's life.

As a safeguard, two doctors must verify that a patient's condition is terminal, and that the patient is capable, is acting voluntarily, and has made an informed decision. If either doctor believes the patient suffers from depression or another psychological disorder that might impair judgment, the patient must be referred for counseling. The patient cannot receive the drugs necessary to

What is a Terminal Condition?

A terminal condition is an irreversible condition that, without life-sustaining procedures, will result in death in the near future or a state of permanent unconsciousness from which recovery is unlikely. Examples of terminal conditions are some types of advanced cancers, irreversible damage to the heart from a heart attack, some types of head injury, and multiple organ failure syndrome. A doctor, usually in consultation with at least one other doctor, makes the determination of a terminal condition.

end life until the counselor determines that the patient is no longer impaired by a psychological illness.

The Oregon Death with Dignity Act is very controversial. It was passed by the narrowest of margins and opponents continue to try to have the law repealed. The ACS has taken a longstanding position against doctor-assisted suicide because it violates one of the most basic doctrines of medical practice: do no harm. Therefore, the ACS opposes the Oregon Death with Dignity Act. In fact, a number of the ACS offices have actively and consistently opposed state-based measures that would permit assisted suicide in their respective states. Patients in pain disproportionately seek out doctor-assisted suicide in Oregon and even in states where the practice is illegal. To deal with this major health concern, the ACS must be highly vigilant in increasing access to pain and symptom management and ensure that no further barriers are established to limit access to essential care.

Research shows that untreated or undertreated pain is often a major factor in a patient's decision to take a life-ending action. Pain need not be a reason to consider ending life because it can be successfully relieved in almost all people with cancer or other serious illnesses. The assurance of adequate pain and symptom management will not only improve the quality of life for people with cancer, but will prevent requests for physician-assisted suicide. Forty-six percent of patients requesting doctor-assisted suicide in Oregon since November 1997 decided not to end their lives once they had been provided adequate pain relief. This demonstrates the need for actively addressing pain and symptom management.

The Impact of the Pain Relief Promotion Act on the Quality of Care for People with Cancer

At the federal level, several members of Congress have introduced legislation addressing a variety of issues related to pain management. In 1999, the Conquering Pain Act was introduced, which offered to provide for a public response to the public health crisis of pain. No action has been taken on the bill thus far.

Another federal piece of legislation considered by Congress has had the potential for impacting how health care professionals treat patients who are in pain, including those with cancer. The Pain Relief Promotion Act (PRPA) was introduced to Congress in 1999, but has not yet been passed (as of the time of this printing). If passed into law, it would affect the lives not only of people in pain but of how health care professionals treat pain. The goal of the PRPA is to promote pain management without permitting doctors to participate in assisted suicide or euthanasia. It was written to override the Death with Dignity Act, however, the legislation could have unintended, but serious negative consequences for the management of pain and palliative care.

The PRPA would ban the use of federally controlled substances (such as opioids) for doctor-assisted suicide and place the responsibility of determining what is considered legitimate medical practice using controlled substances with the Drug Enforcement Agency (DEA). The bill also includes provisions relating to pain management and health professional education and training in an attempt to clarify the important need for pain and symptom management.

Under the PRPA, all doctors, particularly those who care for people with terminal illnesses, will be made especially vulnerable to having their pain management decisions questioned by law enforcement officials who are not qualified to judge the validity of medical decisions. This can result in unnecessary investigation and further disincentives to aggressively treat pain.

The PRPA would give the DEA power to judge the intent of a doctor who uses pain medications. Determining a doctor's intent is very difficult for those without a medical background, particularly for doctors in an area of medicine where effective dosage levels for patients often vary widely from patient to patient. The question of deciding intent should remain in the hands of those properly trained to make such decisions—the medical community and state medical boards. In 2000, the PRPA Act was amended to hold harmless any doctor who treats a patient's pain even if death occurs, and the measure attempts to create a "safe harbor" provision in an effort to shield doctors whose use of federally-controlled drugs unintentionally hasten or cause death. However, this provision does not change the fact that the DEA would explicitly be charged with overseeing the medical use of controlled substances, resulting in a negative impact on cancer pain treatment.

While the PRPA contains positive provisions that directly address pain and symptom management, the ACS maintains that any benefit they may provide would not outweigh the potential threat posed by the bill and that the results could seriously hamper the efforts of doctors to provide adequate pain management.

The ACS respects the right of patients to refuse therapy and the right to request that treatments be withheld or withdrawn, particularly if it dramatically interferes with a person's quality of life. The ACS also has a clear and long-standing position opposing assisted suicide and believes that pain should not be a reason to consider life terminating approaches to end suffering. The ACS recognizes advances must be made in efforts to ensure high-quality pain management and end-of-life care for individuals with cancer. The PRPA would heighten doctors' perceived fear of investigation concerning the prescription of controlled substances for pain and symptom management, which would likely lead to greater undertreatment of pain. Studies have shown that even the perceived threat of investigation leads to undertreatment of pain. Doctors' fear of regulatory scrutiny and criminal penalties, coupled with inadequate knowledge of pain assessment and management, pose looming barriers in ensuring patients adequate treatment of pain caused by cancer or the treatment of cancer. In addition, the PRPA does not comprehensively address the needs of health care professionals, patients, or families for ongoing support and education to counter the current problem of undertreatment of pain—a problem that often leads to requests for doctor-assisted suicide.

The ACS has concluded that as currently written, the PRPA would ban the use of federally controlled substances for doctor-assisted suicide at the expense of controlling pain and advancing symptom management. These issues are both critically important, but are separate issues. While the ACS opposes all patient deaths stemming from assisted suicides, heavier weight must be given to the more than 1,500 individuals who die of cancer every day in this country—more than half of whom die in pain unnecessarily. Moreover, the ACS believes that the best approach to help cancer patients prevent assisted suicide is through the adoption of active policies and the provision of resources to prevent and ease pain and suffering in people with cancer, especially those near the end-of-life.

Advocating for Change

By being an advocate for cancer and supporting legislation that supports cancer research and care of people with cancer, you can effect change and make valuable contributions to the fight against the disease. Advocates are making great progress in the legislative battle against cancer, but there's still a long way to go. Each year more than 10,000 cancer-related proposals are introduced before Congress and state legislatures, but only a small number become law. In order to eliminate cancer as a major health concern, the number of cancer-related laws passed must grow.

WHAT YOU CAN DO

To ensure that our lawmakers and policymakers pass measures that will help us better prevent and find a cure for cancer in our lifetime, organizations like the ACS monitor cancer-related legislative and policy efforts. Its grassroots advocacy network currently consists of more than 125,000 members who receive a monthly national newsletter and state-specific advocacy and legislative information. Programs like the ACS's Campaign Against Cancer seek to educate political candidates and representatives about the issues surrounding cancer, and also to understand what voters think about these issues.

The ACS offers other opportunities as well. For example, you may serve as an advocate for the ACS or serve as a media spokesperson on important cancer-related issues. You may be able to assist in the creation and passage of legislative measures that affect people with cancer and their care. Volunteers may contact state and federal senators and representatives to discuss important cancer-related topics and to campaign for the passage of important laws that affect people with cancer. Volunteers are needed to share their stories and demonstrate to the public the important role of research and other programs.

Lawmakers and policymakers need to know how many and how substantially their actions touch people with cancer and their loved ones. As an advocate, you can work with elected officials and national and community leaders to secure funding for cancer research; or for programs that heighten cancer awareness and improve prevention, screening, detection and follow-up care; and to ensure timely, quality cancer care for those who need it.

What can you do to sway public policy and move cancer prevention, research, and control forward? These are the most effective ways the ACS can secure funding and support for research and programs so desperately needed in the war against cancer.

- Communicate regularly with your lawmakers and key policymakers to make sure they pay attention to cancer-related issues.

Sample Letter to a Legislator

Here is an example of a letter urging a senator to vote for a bill. Your letter should include your views on the issue and how the bill affects you, your family, or your community, for example.

The Honorable Mary Johnson
Senate Office Building
Washington, DC 20510

Dear Senator Johnson:

As someone who lives and votes in your district, I am writing to urge you to support the [*insert the name of the legislation you're writing about*] Act [*insert House or Senate bill number*]. This legislation has the ability to directly impact the lives of those living with cancer and the millions of others who will have cancer in the future.

[*Insert a paragraph about why this issue is important to you. You may want to state personal reasons. Avoid making the letter sound like a form letter. Explain how the issue will affect you, your family, your business, or an organization you belong to. State how the issue will affect your community, state, and nation.*]

As a constituent and someone concerned about cancer, I urge you to help stop the toll cancer takes on America by supporting [*insert bill number*]. I would very much like to know your position on this legislation and when you think it will come up for debate. Please know how important this issue is to me and likely thousands of other cancer-concerned citizens in our community.

I will monitor this and other cancer-related votes carefully throughout this Congress.

Thank you for your time and attention.
[Your typed name]
[Your signature]

- Let them know that cancer research and treatment and prevention programs are critical concerns to you.
- Keep cancer issues in the media by writing letters to the editor for newspapers and by participating in television or radio call-in shows.
- Talk about the issues, and encourage others to join the fight.

Contact Your Lawmakers

To find out what is currently in legislation and how to contact your legislators, you can begin by searching the ACS web site (www.cancer.org). Here you'll find information about the following:

- Important Issues and Legislation—Important issues in current bills and legislative alerts.
- Guide to Congress—Congress members listed by name, state, committee, or leadership directory.
- Write to Congress—Enter your ZIP Code and click "search" to receive information on how to contact your Representative.
- Congress Today—Schedules for the House and Senate, plus searchable committee schedules.

Keep Cancer Issues in the Media Spotlight

Keeping the media interested in covering cancer ensures that a healthy discussion of prevention, detection, education, and research takes place and that the topic remains a societal priority. You can help by writing letters to the editor of your local newspaper about cancer-related issues and by participating in radio and television call-in programs. As a newspaper or magazine subscriber or member of a television audience, your letters and phone calls carry weight and achieve results.

Support Cancer-Related Initiatives

The ACS and other organizations work on many fronts to fight cancer, from laboratory research for innovative cancer treatments to helping patients get to a doctor's appointment and supporting organizations that help people avoid and overcome cancer. Challenge lawmakers and policymakers to adopt public policies that affect cancer outcomes and improve health care initiatives. Among our priorities, the ACS:

- Seeks to protect medical records and advocate for privacy laws while respecting the need for data for life-saving research.
- Works to ensure any Medicare reform proposal meets the needs of people with cancer.
- Studies ways to better investigate alternative therapies.
- Encourages support for palliative care and hospice services.
- Seeks to improve quality-of-life and end-of-life care and helps people with cancer understand what options they have if their cancer progresses.
- Advances programs to encourage physical activity and curb poor nutrition.

Talk About the Issues and Encourage Others to Join the Fight

Tell your family, friends, and coworkers about cancer-related legislation and encourage them to get involved in supporting the passage of important laws. Start a telephone "phone tree" or an e-mail list to alert friends and coworkers as cancer-related legislation moves through the process.

Your efforts are needed to educate lawmakers about issues that are important to you, the voter. You have the power to make cancer a lawmaker's priority. Attend town meetings and candidate forums; talk to the candidates when they are in your community; and follow what your local newspapers and television and radio stations are reporting on cancer issues. This will teach candidates how important it is to our country to defeat cancer. If you want to show lawmakers—from the President down—that they need to make the fight against cancer a national priority, begin by researching involvement in activist organizations that are fighting for the specific causes you believe in. You can also go to the ACS web site and click on Take Action to learn more about ACS efforts and the ACS Action Network.

The Advance Directive

People's rights to make decisions regarding their own health care and the conditions under which they want medical treatment continued or discontinued are recognized under both the U.S. Constitution and state laws. Competent adults have the right to refuse or accept medical treatments, even those that will save or prolong their lives. This right is sometimes called "autonomy" to make decisions about one's own health care. However, if a person is unable to make medical

End-of-Life Care

End-of-life decisions are those that patients make about how they wish to be cared for and treated when they are dying. End-of-life decisions can include whether to accept or refuse life-sustaining treatments. The initiation or withdrawal of life-saving or life-preserving measures is a tremendously sensitive topic. End-of-life care and related decisions spark deep emotional reactions among patients, families, and health care professionals. Patients and loved ones may be better able to sort out and understand conflicting beliefs or desires and to clarify the goals of care by speaking with a trusted medical professional or counselor.

If you are a caregiver considering whether to begin or end life-sustaining interventions for a patient who is incapable of making the decision, it is crucial and ethical to consider all of the potential impacts, both positive and negative, that the choices will have on the patient. Always consider the patient's point of view when possible.

decisions because of a temporary or permanent illness or injury, the person still has the right to refuse or accept treatment. One way to maintain this right is to express your wishes about future health care choices ahead of time in what is called an advance directive.

An advance directive is a legal document that states one's wishes about health care choices or that designates someone to make those choices if a person becomes unable to do so. An advance directive can be simple or complex. In other words, it can be general in nature with minimal direction about care, or it can be very specific, detailing wishes regarding acceptance or refusal of all types of life-sustaining treatments. A statement can also be included about organ and tissue donation.

Advance directives can only be used for decisions about medical care. Other people cannot use them to control one's money or property. An advance directive takes effect only when people are unable to make their own decisions. Others can make health care decisions for a person without an advance directive, but there is greater assurance that wishes will be carried out with a written advance directive.

All people who receive medical care in hospitals, enroll in health plans, and enter into hospice or home-care agreements must be given written information about their rights under their state's law to make decisions about medical care, including the right to accept or refuse medical or surgical treatment. In addition, everyone must be given information about their rights to make advance directives. Remember that every person's circumstances differ and that laws about advance directives vary from state to state.

TYPES OF ADVANCE DIRECTIVES

One way to communicate your own end-of-life decisions based on your values and priorities while you are competent to do so is through an advance directive. The two most common types of advance directives are the living will and the power of attorney for health care.

The Living Will

A living will is a document that directs medical personnel to provide or withhold certain types of medical treatment, such as life-sustaining procedures or artificial life support. It usually states that life-sustaining measures should be withheld or withdrawn if a person is terminally ill or near death and unable to make these decisions.

Copies of a living will should be given to trusted loved ones or family members, as well as to your doctor, nurse, hospital, and anyone else who is caring for you. You can change or cancel a living will at any time.

A living will is usually more limited in its scope than a power of attorney, covering fewer conditions and treatments (see below). A living will is also not as powerful as a power of attorney for health care because it contains only written instructions; no one is named to interpret the document or to ensure that the wishes are carried out.

Power of Attorney for Health Care

Another form of advance directive is the power of attorney for health care (often called the durable power of attorney). The power of attorney is a legal document that identifies a proxy for the patient. This is someone specifically chosen by the patient as a surrogate decision-maker to speak for the patient in any health-related situation in which the patient is no longer able to make decisions.

What is Life-Sustaining Medical Treatment?

Life-sustaining medical treatment is defined differently from state-to-state. In general, life-sustaining medical treatment is any mechanical or artificial means that sustains, restores, or substitutes for a vital body function and which would prolong the dying process for a terminally ill patient. Life-sustaining medical treatment may consist of some or all of the following: cardiopulmonary resuscitation (CPR), artificial respiration (mouth-to-mouth breathing, manual ventilation, or a ventilator), medications to artificially alter blood pressure and heart function, artificial nutrition/hydration, dialysis, and certain surgical procedures (amputation, feeding tube placement, removal of tumor, organ transplant). Nutrition/hydration (food and water) are not usually defined as life-sustaining unless they are provided by a feeding tube or intravenous line. Medications or procedures necessary to provide comfort or ease pain are not usually considered life-sustaining procedures, but rather comfort measures.

This person, also called an agent, negotiates on the patient's behalf with doctors and caregivers and is required to make decisions according to the patient's directions. In a health care power of attorney, individuals can indicate the specific kinds of treatments or procedures that they do or do not want. If wishes are not known for a particular situation, the agent will make decisions based on what they think a person would want and what is in the person's best interest. The scope of the agent's authority can also be limited.

The agent should be someone the patient trusts to carry out his or her wishes. The patient should also name an alternate agent just in case the primary agent becomes unable or unwilling to act on the patient's behalf. The law does not allow the agent to be a doctor, nurse, or other person providing health care to the person on the date the power of attorney for health care is signed unless that person is a close relative.

Power of attorney may be limited to health decisions, but it can also be expanded to allow an agent to act on your behalf in money matters. This may mean paying your bills or signing your name on financial transactions. Copies of the power of attorney should be given to your executor or attorney. A copy also should be given to the person granted the power of attorney and to your agent. A copy also can be placed in a safe deposit box.

LAWS RELATED TO ADVANCE DIRECTIVES

All states and the District of Columbia recognize and have laws concerning advance directives. However, state laws vary considerably so the exact names of documents, restrictions, and formalities also vary geographically.

Most states have advance directive forms that are specific to the laws of that state, but most states do not require that a specific form be used. In some states, the language in the forms can be changed to reflect personal values, priorities, and wishes. Some forms have checklists that make it easy to specify your choices. Forms for advance directives can usually be obtained from state bar associations or the American Bar Association (see Resources).

The requirements for creating advance directives are generally similar from state to state. The minimum age is usually the age that the state uses to define a person as an adult. All states require that at least one person of adult age not related by blood, marriage, or adoption witness the signature and date on the advance directive. Some states require two witnesses. A notary public may serve as one witness.

There are oral advance directives and mental health directives. An oral advance directive is a spoken statement made by a person who is physically ill and unable to obtain a living will or power of attorney for health care, and is written by another person (e.g., a doctor) and properly witnessed. Several states recognize such statements as formal advance directives. A mental health directive allows the patient a choice regarding treatment if he or she should become seriously mentally ill and cannot make health care decisions.

The Patient Self-Determination Act

The Patient Self-Determination Act (PSDA) was passed in 1990, and became effective on December 1, 1991. The PSDA encourages the public to make choices and decisions ab out the types and extent of medical care they want to accept or refuse in the future, should they be unable due to illness to make those decisions. The PSDA requires all health care agencies (hospitals, long-term care facilities, home health agencies) receiving Medicare and Medicaid reimbursement to recognize the living will and power of attorney for health care as advance directives.

How to Write an Advance Directive

- **Learn all you can about advance directives before you begin.** Know your rights and the laws pertaining to advance directives in your state. See the Resources section at the back of the book for contact information of places to go for help about creating living wills and power of attorney. Call the ACS for more information about advance directives and frequently asked questions about this topic.

- **Decide whether you want to write a living will and/or a power of attorney for health care.** Understand the meanings and the differences between the two documents. The power of attorney for health care provides greater assurance that your wishes will be followed.

- **Decide on the content of your advance directive.** Be specific about your wishes regarding specific medical interventions, such as cardiopulmonary resuscitation (CPR), artificial respiration, medications to make your heart function, kidney dialysis, artificial feeding (tube or intravenous), and surgical procedures.

- **Discuss your decision and wishes with family members, close friends, doctors, and an attorney.** Communicating your end-of-life decisions to those close to you will help ensure that your wishes are carried out.

The PSDA did not create new rights for patients, but reaffirmed the common-law right of self-determination as guaranteed by the Fourteenth Amendment. Under the PSDA, health care agencies must ask patients whether they have an advance directive and provide them with educational materials about their rights under state law.

Discussing these matters is difficult for all parties involved and can generate deep emotional responses. Yet for patients to know that their wishes will be respected and followed can also bring a sense of peace, closure, and emotional healing for themselves as well as families and friends.

- **Choose your health care proxy or surrogate decision-maker.** This is one of the most important decisions you will ever make. Choose this person carefully. It should be someone that you trust and believe will ensure that your wishes are followed even if they include denying life-sustaining treatments. Your proxy, or agent, will have the power to carry out your wishes if and when you become unable to express them yourself because of your medical condition. Have one or more witnesses sign your advance directive and give a copy of the document to your health care proxy. Discuss your advance directive periodically with your proxy so that important responsibilities remain clear.

- **Keep a copy of your advance directive in a readily accessible place.** Make sure that someone close to you knows where a copy of your advance directive is at all times in the event that you are unable to retrieve it yourself. You may also want to give a copy to your attorney.

Appendix A

Cancer Pain Drug Information

NONOPIOIDS (for mild to moderate pain)				
Drug Type	**Generic Name and (Trade Name)**	**Action (Use)**	**Delivery Method**	**Side Effects**
Antipyretic (fever reducing) Analgesic	acetaminophen (Acephen, Actamin, Anacin-3, Apacet, Anesin, Dapa, Datril, Genapap, Genebs, Gentabs, Halenol, Liquiprin, Meda Cap, Panadol, Panex, Suppap, Tempra, Tenol, Ty Caps, Tylenol)	-relieves pain, decreases pain perception -reduces fever	-oral -rectal	*More Common:* -None *Less Common:* -possible liver damage in those who consume three or more alcoholic drinks a day, or in those with liver or kidney disease -few side effects when taken as directed
Nonsteroidal anti-inflammatory drug (NSAID)	aspirin, acetylsalicyclic acid (ASA, Aspergum, Bayer aspirin, Easprin, Ecotrin, Empirin)	-decreases pain perception -reduces inflammation -reduces fever -relieves pain	-oral -rectal	*More Common:* -increased bleeding time -heartburn -increased bruising -sweating *Less Common:* -bleeding in gastrointestinal tract -flushing -ringing in the ears -hearing loss -dizziness
NSAID	ibuprofen (Advil, Genpril, Haltran, Ibuprin, Midol 200, Nuprin, Rufen)	-decreases pain perception -reduces inflammation -reduces fever -relieves pain	-oral	*More Common:* -dizziness -heartburn -nausea -drowsiness *Less Common:* -vomiting -constipation -loss of appetite -diarrhea -sores in mouth or on lips -bloating -abdominal pain -bleeding from the gastrointestinal tract -headache -nervousness -fatigue -anxiety -confusion -depression -mood swings -peptic ulcers

Drug Type	Generic Name and (Trade Name)	Action (Use)	Delivery Method	Side Effects
NSAID	salsalate (Disalcid, Salsalate, Salflex)	-decreases pain perception -reduces inflammation -reduces fever	-oral	*More Common:* -dizziness *Less Common:* -nausea -heartburn -loss of appetite -increased risk of peptic ulcer -ringing in the ears -vomiting -diarrhea -confusion -lethargy -headache -sweating
NSAID	choline magnesium trisalicylate (Trilisate)	-decreases pain perception -reduces inflammation -reduces fever	-oral	*More Common:* -None *Less Common:* -flushing -dizziness -decreased hearing -ringing in the ears
NSAID	celecoxib (Celebrex)	-decreases pain perception -reduces inflammation	-oral	*More Common:* -abdominal pain -diarrhea -indigestion -gas -nausea -back pain -edema in the extremities -dizziness -headache -inability to sleep -sore throat -runny nose -rash *Less Common:* -constipation -difficulty swallowing -gastroenteritis -acid reflux -vomiting -chest pain -increased blood pressure -allergic reaction -rash -flu-like symptoms -leg cramps -migraine -ringing in the ears -change in liver and kidney function -problems with blood clotting -difficulty with urination

Drug Type	Generic Name and (Trade Name)	Action (Use)	Delivery Method	Side Effects
NSAID	diclofenac (Voltaren)	-decreases pain perception -reduces inflammation	-oral	*More Common:* -nausea -vomiting -heartburn -gastrointestinal bleeding -headache -dizziness -changes in liver function -diarrhea -constipation -rash -itching -ringing in the ears *Less Common:* -swelling of lips and tongue -allergic reaction -increased blood pressure -congestive heart failure -vomiting -yellow skin -anemia -inability to sleep -drowsiness -depression -anxiety -double or blurred vision -irritability -nose bleed -asthma -chest pain -bruising -tingling -frequent urination
NSAID	diflunisal (Dolobid)	-decreases pain perception -reduces inflammation	-oral	*More Common:* -abdominal pain -constipation -diarrhea -dizziness -fatigue -headache -inability to sleep -indigestion -nausea -rash -ringing in ears -sleepiness -vomiting *Less Common:* -gastrointestinal bleeding -anemia -blurred vision -confusion -depression -disorientation -dry mouth and nose

Drug Type	Generic Name and (Trade Name)	Action (Use)	Delivery Method	Side Effects
NSAID	diflunisal (Dolobid) cont'd			-fluid retention -flushing -changes in liver function -hives -inflammation of lips and tongue -itching -changes in kidney function -light-headedness -loss of appetite -nervousness -gastric ulcer -tingling in the extremities -protein or blood in urine, difficulty urinating
NSAID	fenoprofen (Nalfon)	-decreases pain perception -reduces inflammation	-oral	*More Common:* -indigestion -nausea -constipation -vomiting -abdominal pain -diarrhea -headache -drowsiness -dizziness -sweating -ringing in the ears -blurred vision -palpitations -nervousness -tingling -swelling in the extremities -shortness of breath -fatigue *Less Common:* -gastritis -peptic ulcer with and without perforation -gastrointestinal bleeding -loss of appetite -gas -dry mouth -change in liver function -change in kidney function -allergic reaction -bruising
NSAID	ketoprofen (Orudis)	-decreases pain perception -reduces inflammation	-oral	*More Common:* -indigestion -nausea -vomiting -diarrhea -constipation -headache -dizziness -drowsiness

Drug Type	Generic Name and (Trade Name)	Action (Use)	Delivery Method	Side Effects
NSAID	ketoprofen (Orudis) cont'd			-depression -anxiety -ringing in the ears -rash -visual disturbances -change in renal function *Less Common:* -gastrointestinal bleeding -increased blood pressure and heart rate -change in liver function -bleeding problems -muscle pain -confusion -migraine -shortness of breath -sweating -rash
NSAID	piroxicam (Feldene)	-decreases pain perception -reduces inflammation -reduces fever	-oral	*More Common:* -swelling of the extremities -nausea -heartburn -gastric ulcers -gastointestinal bleeding -diarrhea -ringing in the ears -drowsiness -nervousness -dry mouth -abnormal kidney function *Less Common:* -changes in liver function -allergic reaction -rash -itching -depression -increased blood sugar -anemia -dizziness -headache -asthma -increased blood pressure
NSAID	indomethacin (Indocin)	-decreases pain perception -reduces inflammation -reduces fever	-oral	*More Common:* -headache -vomiting -ringing in ears (tinnitus) -tremor -sleeplessness *Less Common:* -dizziness -depression -fatigue -numbness and tingling in hands and/or feet

Drug Type	Generic Name and (Trade Name)	Action (Use)	Delivery Method	Side Effects
NSAID	indomethacin (Indocin) cont'd			-nausea -loss of appetite -heartburn, indigestion, epigastric pain -bleeding from gastrointestinal tract
NSAID	naproxen (Naprosyn)	-decreases pain perception -reduces inflammation	-oral	*More Common:* -constipation -heartburn -abdominal pain -nausea -indigestion -diarrhea -mouth sores -headache -dizziness -drowsiness -itching -rash -sweating -ringing in the ears -swelling of the extremities -shortness of breath *Less Common:* -abnormal liver function -gastrointestinal bleeding and/or perforation -vomiting -yellowing of skin -alteration in kidney function -low platelet count -low white blood cell count -depression -difficulty sleeping -itching -hearing changes -allergic reaction
NSAID	rofecoxib (Vioxx)	-decreases pain perception -reduces inflammation	-oral	*More Common:* -abdominal pain -fatigue -dizziness -flu-like symptoms -swelling in legs -upper respiratory infection -increased blood pressure -indigestion -heartburn -nausea -sinusitis -back pain -headache -bronchitis -urinary tract infection

Drug Type	Generic Name and (Trade Name)	Action (Use)	Delivery Method	Side Effects
NSAID	rofecoxib (Vioxx) cont'd			*Less Common:* -dry mouth -inflammation of the esophagus -gas -acid reflux -allergic reaction -weight gain -increased blood cholesterol -muscle pain -depression -anxiety -asthma -rash -difficulty urinating
NSAID	ketorolac tromethamine (Toradol)	-decreases pain perception -reduces inflammation -reduces fever -only NSAID that can be given by injection	-IV -oral -IM	*More Common:* -heartburn -dizziness -drowsiness -lightheadedness *Less Common:* -nausea -vomiting -loss of appetite -diarrhea -constipation -sores in mouth or on lips -bloating -abdominal pain -peptic ulcers -bleeding from gastrointestinal tract -headache -nervousness -fatigue -anxiety -confusion -depression -mood swings
OPIOIDS (for moderate to severe pain)				
Opioid	codeine -when combined with acetaminophen (Phenaphen with codeine, Tylenol with codeine, Capital with codeine, Vodaphen, Odalan) codeine-when combined with aspirin (Empirin with codeine, Soma Compound with codeine, Fiorinal with codeine)	-relieves mild to moderate pain -alters the perception of pain	-IV -oral -IM*	*More Common:* -nausea -constipation -drowsiness -sedation -mood changes -dizziness -dry mouth *Less Common:* -euphoria -depression -mental clouding -vomiting -dizziness when changing position

*IM route is to be avoided if at all possible

Drug Type	Generic Name and (Trade Name)	Action (Use)	Delivery Method	Side Effects
	codeine cont'd			-flushing -itching -sweating -decreased heart rate -difficulty urinating
Opioid	fentanyl citrate (Actiq)	-relieves moderate to severe pain -alters the perception of pain -used for breakthrough pain or before procedures	-transmucosal: lozenge on a stick/handle, like a lollipop, to be placed between cheek and lower gum	*More Common:* -sleepiness -dizziness -headache -fever -fatigue -constipation *Less Common:* -difficulty breathing -cough -sore throat -sedation -anxiety -confusion -depression -difficulty sleeping -muscle aches -itching -rash -sweating -nausea -vomiting -loss of appetite -heartburn
Opioid	fentanyl transdermal system (Duragesic)	-relieves moderate to severe pain -alters the perception of pain	-skin patch	*More Common:* -sleepiness -dizziness -constipation -nausea *Less Common:* -difficulty breathing -decreased breathing rate -confusion -depression -nervousness -tremors -lack of coordination -euphoria -difficulty speaking -vomiting -chest pain -decreased blood pressure when changing position -sweating -difficulty urinating -rash -itching

Drug Type	Generic Name and (Trade Name)	Action (Use)	Delivery Method	Side Effects
Opioid	hydromorphone (Dilaudid)	-relieves moderate to severe pain -is similar to morphine -alters the perception of pain	-IV -oral -IM*	*More Common:* -constipation -drowsiness -sedation -dizziness -nausea -dry mouth *Less Common:* -mood changes -euphoria -mental clouding -decreased breathing rate -vomiting -delayed digestion -decreased blood pressure when changing position -decreased heart rate
Opioid	levorphanol tartrate (Levo-Dromoran)	-relieves moderate to severe pain -is similar to morphine -alters the perception of pain	-IV -SQ -oral	*More Common:* -constipation -drowsiness -sedation -nausea -dry mouth *Less Common:* -changes in mood -euphoria -depression -mental clouding -decreased rate of breathing -vomiting -delayed digestion -decreased blood pressure when changing position -decreased heart rate
Opioid	meperidine hydrochloride (Demerol); merperidine with promethazine (Mepergan Fortis)	-relieves moderate to severe pain -alters the perception of pain -not an effective choice for chronic cancer pain	-IV -oral -SQ -IM*	*More Common:* -constipation -drowsiness -sedation -nausea -vomiting -dizziness -dry mouth *Less Common:* -changes in mood -euphoria -mental clouding -decreased breathing rate -decreased blood pressure when changing position -delayed digestion -decreased heart rate

*IM route is to be avoided if at all possible

Drug Type	Generic Name and (Trade Name)	Action (Use)	Delivery Method	Side Effects
Opioid	methadone (Dolophine, Methadose)	-relieves moderate to severe pain -alters the perception of pain	-SQ -oral -IM*	*More Common:* -constipation -drowsiness -sedation -nausea -dizziness -dry mouth *Less Common:* -vomiting -changes in mood -euphoria -depression -mental clouding -decreased breathing rate -decreased blood pressure when changing position -delayed digestion -decreased heart rate
Opioid	morphine (Astramorph, Duramorph, Infumorph, Kadian, Morphine Sulfate Sustained Release, MS Contin, MSIR, Oramorph, Roxanol)	-relieves moderate to severe pain -alters the perception of pain	-IV -SQ -by infusion -rectal -into spinal canal	*More Common:* -constipation -drowsiness -sedation -nausea -dizziness -dry mouth *Less Common:* -vomiting -changes in mood -euphoria -depression -mental clouding -decreased breathing rate -decreased blood pressure when changing position -delayed digestion -decreased heart rate
Opioid	oxycodone (OxyContin, Roxicodone); oxycodone with aspirin (Percodan, Endodan, Roxiprin); oxycodone with acetaminophen (Percocet)	-relieves moderate to severe pain -alters the perception of pain	-oral	*More Common:* -constipation -drowsiness -sedation -nausea -dizziness -dry mouth *Less Common:* -vomiting -changes in mood -euphoria -depression -mental clouding -decreased breathing rate -decreased blood pressure when changing position -delayed digestion -decreased heart rate

*IM route is to be avoided if at all possible

ADJUVANT ANALGESICS (antianxiety drugs, anticonvulsants, antidepressants, steroids)				
Drug Type	**Generic Name and (Trade Name)**	**Action (Use)**	**Delivery Method**	**Side Effects**
Antianxiety	buspirone hydrochloride (Buspar)	-action not known, but it affects the neurotransmitters in the brain that bring about the feeling of anxiety	-oral	*More Common:* -None *Less Common:* -dizziness -drowsiness -headache
Antianxiety	alprazolam (Xanax)	-reduces anxiety -muscle relaxant -anticonvulsant effects	-oral	*More Common:* -dry mouth -decreased mental alertness *The following side effects occur when first starting the drug:* -drowsiness -fatigue -lethargy -weakness -confusion -headache *Less Common:* -nausea -vomiting -change in body weight
Antianxiety	clonazepam (Klonopin)	-manages anxiety, panic attacks, seizures, involuntary movements	-oral	*More Common:* -drowsiness *Less Common:* -decrease in blood pressure when changing position -decreased mental alertness -dizziness
Antianxiety	diazepam (Valium)	-reduces anxiety -causes muscle relaxation -prevents seizures	-IV -oral -IM*	*More Common:* *The following side effects occur when first starting the drug:* -drowsiness -feeling tired -confusion -headache *Less Common:* -feeling "hung over" the next day -decreased coordination -decreased mental alertness -decreased in blood pressure -decreased heart rate
Antianxiety	lorazepam (Ativan)	-reduces anxiety -causes muscle relaxation -prevents seizures -decreases chance of nausea and vomiting following chemotherapy -causes amnesia	-IV -oral -SQ -IM	*More Common:* *The following side effects occur when first starting the drug:* -drowsiness -fatigue -confusion -weakness -headache

*IM route is to be avoided if at all possible

Drug Type	Generic Name and (Trade Name)	Action (Use)	Delivery Method	Side Effects
Anitianxiety	lorazepam (Ativan) cont'd			*Less Common:* -nausea -dry mouth -constipation -lack of coordination -decreased mental alertness -change in heart rate -change in blood pressure
Antianxiety	oxazepam (Serax)	-reduces anxiety -muscle relaxation -prevention of seizures	-oral	*More Common:* -drowsiness -fatigue -weakness -dry mouth -constipation *Less Common:* -nausea -vomiting -change in weight -lack of coordination -decreased mental alertness
Antinausea Antivomiting Antianxiety	haloperidol (Haldol)	-prevents nausea and vomiting resulting from chemotherapy -decreases agitation	-oral -IM[*]	*More Common:* -feeling sedated -sleepiness *Less Common:* -decreased breathing rate -increased heart rate -decrease in blood pressure when changing position
Anticonvulsant	gabapentin (Neurontin)	-helpful in treating neuropathic pain	-oral	*More Common:* -sleepiness -dizziness -fatigue *Less Common:* -difficulty walking -tremor -nervousness -difficulty speaking -amnesia -depression -decreased muscle coordination -headache -confusion -mood swings -numbness in hands and/or feet -decreased reflexes -irritability -heartburn -nausea -vomiting -rash -hair thinning

[*]IM route is to be avoided if at all possible

Drug Type	Generic Name and (Trade Name)	Action (Use)	Delivery Method	Side Effects
Antidepressant	doxepin hydrochloride (Sinequan)	-decreases or stops the feeling of depression	-oral	*More Common:* -drowsiness *Less Common:* -dry mouth -decreased appetite -indigestion -changes in taste including metallic taste of foods -urinary retention
Antidepressant	nefazodone hydrochloride (Serzone)	-prevents or relieves depression	-oral	*More Common:* -dizziness -drowsiness -difficulty sleeping -dry mouth -nausea -constipation -headache -feeling "blah" *Less Common:* -lightheadedness -heartburn
Antidepressant	trazodone hydrochloride (Desyrel, Trialodine)	-decreases feeling of depression	-oral	*More Common:* -drowsiness -dizziness -lightheadedness -decrease in blood pressure when changing from a lying or sitting position to standing *Less Common:* -fatigue -nightmares -confusion -anger -excitement -decreased mental concentration -disorientation -nervousness -difficulty remembering
Antidepressant	venlafaxine hydrochloride (Effexor)	-prevents or relieves the feeling of depression	-oral	*More Common:* -migraine headache -dizziness when standing up -tightness in the jaw -nausea *Less Common:* -loss of appetite -constipation -problem in sexual function -feeling "blah" -neck pain -hang-over like effect -bone pain -black and blue spots on the skin -problem urinating

Drug Type	Generic Name and (Trade Name)	Action (Use)	Delivery Method	Side Effects
Antidepressant-Selective Serotonin Reuptake Inhibitor (SSRI)	fluoxetine hydrochloride (Prozac)	-decreases the feeling of depression	-oral	More Common: -headache Less Common: -difficulty speaking -anxiety -decreased ability to concentrate -tremor -dizziness -nausea -loss of appetite -weight loss in underweight individuals -muscle or bone pain
Antidepressant-Selective Serotonin Reuptake Inhibitor (SSRI)	paroxetine hydrochloride (Paxil)	-decreases the feeling of depression	-oral	More Common: -sweating Less Common: -sleepiness -dizziness -difficulty sleeping -tremor -nervousness -feeling "blah" -nausea -decreased appetite -decreased sexual ability
Antidepressant-Tricyclic	amitriptyline hydrochloride (Elavil)	-prevents and relieves depression -reduces peripheral nerve pain	-oral	More Common: -drowsiness -dizziness -weakness -lethargy -fatigue -dry mouth Less Common: -confusion (especially in the elderly) -disorientation -hallucinations -decreased blood pressure when changing position -increased heart rate -increased blood pressure -loss of appetite -nausea -vomiting -diarrhea -urinary retention
Antidepressant-Tricyclic	desipramine hydrochloride (Norpramin, Pertofrane)	-prevents or relieves depression -reduces pain related to peripheral neuropathy	-oral	More Common: -drowsiness -dizziness -weakness -fatigue -dry mouth

Drug Type	Generic Name and (Trade Name)	Action (Use)	Delivery Method	Side Effects
Antidepressant-Tricyclic	desipramine hydrochloride (Norpramin, Pertofrane) cont'd			Less Common: -confusion (especially in the elderly) -disorientation -hallucinations -decrease in blood pressure when changing position -increased heart rate -loss of appetite -urinary retention
Antidepressant-Tricyclic	imipramine pamoate (Tofranil-PM)	-decreases or stops the feeling of depression -promotes sleep -treats hiccups	-oral -IM*	More Common: -drowsiness -dizziness -weakness -fatigue Less Common: -confusion -disorientation -change in blood pressure when changing position -increased heart rate -dry mouth -decreased appetite -nausea -urinary retention
Antidepressant-Tricyclic	nortriptyline hydrochloride (Aventyl, Pamelor)	-decreases feeling of depression -increases pain relief from narcotic drugs	-oral	More Common: -drowsiness -fatigue -dizziness -dry mouth -vomiting -diarrhea -abdominal cramping Less Common: -confusion -disorientation -nausea -changes in appetite -urinary retention
Corticosteroid	prednisone (Apo-prednisone, Deltasone, Orasone, Prednisone)	-decreases inflammation	-oral	More Common: -delayed wound healing -mood changes -depression -increased blood sugar -increased appetite with weight gain -bruising of the skin -sleep disturbance -increased risk of infection -sodium and fluid retention with swelling in ankles, increased blood pressure, and congestive heart failure

*IM route is to be avoided if at all possible

Drug Type	Generic Name and (Trade Name)	Action (Use)	Delivery Method	Side Effects
Corticosteroid	prednisone (Apo-prednisone, Deltasone, Orasone, Prednisone) cont'd			*Less Common:* -decreased blood potassium level (symptoms are loss of appetite, muscle twitching, increased thirst, increased urination) -weakness -fracture of weak bones -fungal infections (white patches in mouth, vagina) -sweating -diarrhea -nausea -headache -increased heart rate -loss of calcium from bones
Corticosteroid	dexamethasone (Decadron)	-relieves nausea associated with chemotherapy -reduces swelling of the brain	-IV -oral	*More Common:* -increased appetite -irritation of stomach -euphoria -difficulty sleeping -mood changes -flushing -increased blood sugar -decreased blood potassium level *Less Common:* -depression -headache -sweating -increased blood pressure

Appendix B

Guidelines for Pain Management

In recent years, more attention has focused on the issue of cancer pain. Professional nurse, physician, and health care organizations have developed standards for education, training, and patient care to ensure that people with cancer pain are receiving appropriate care. Below are some of the current pain control guidelines for health professionals and hospitals that are used to help guide care for people with cancer.

JOINT COMMISSION ON THE ACCREDITATION OF HEALTHCARE ORGANIZATIONS

The Joint Commission on the Accreditation of Healthcare Organizations (JCAHO), taking a major step toward addressing issues related to pain control, issued pain management guidelines that took effect January 1, 2001. The JCAHO is the agency that is responsible for accrediting hospitals, ambulatory care centers, some long-term care centers, and other facilities where people go for medical treatment. Although the standards do not outline exactly what medications doctors are to prescribe, they do provide formal acknowledgment of pain, a way to measure it, and a requirement that it be recorded in the patient's medical record. The guidelines are important because they require that health professional document a patient's level of pain. While in the hospital, patients will be asked to rate their pain at all stages of treatment using a numerical scale, so it can be tracked and attended to regularly. And, hospitals will be rated on their compliance with these guidelines. The standards, available on the JCAHO web site (http://www.jcaho.org/standards_frm.html), require accredited facilities to:

- Recognize the patient's right to pain assessment and management.
- Assess, or evaluate, the existence, nature, and intensity of pain in all patients.
- Record assessment results in a way that facilitates regular reassessment and follow-up.
- Make sure staff members are competent at assessing and managing pain, and address the issue in orientation of new staff.

- Set policies and procedures for the appropriate prescribing and ordering of pain medications.
- Educate patients and families about effective pain management.
- Address patients' pain management needs when they are discharged from the facility.

AGENCY FOR HEALTHCARE RESEARCH AND QUALITY

The Agency for Healthcare Research and Quality (AHRQ), an office within the U.S. Department of Health and Human Services, is responsible for supporting research to improve the quality of health care, reduce its cost, and broaden access to needed services. One of AHRQ's highest priorities is providing consumers with science-based, easily understandable information that will help them make informed decisions about their own personal health care. They offer a number of clinical practice guidelines on common health problems in consumer versions for the public. These guidelines are written by a panel of private-sector experts sponsored by what was then the Agency for Health Care Policy and Research. The latest consumer version of the *Clinical Practice Guideline on Management of Cancer Pain*, published in March 1994, is entitled, *Managing Cancer Pain*. To order a copy of this booklet, call AHRQ at 800-358-9295, or access them via their web site at http://www.ahrq.gov (see Resources).

The AHRQ pain management guidelines emphasize the importance of:

- A collaborative, interdisciplinary approach to pain control involving all members of the health care team, the patient, and family.
- Frequent reassessment of the patient's pain.
- Use of drug and nondrug pain control strategies.
- A formal, institutionalized approach to managing pain, with clear lines of responsibility.

These guidelines include strategies for pain control in general as well as for specific types of cancer pain, address issues of pain control in specific groups, and contain a range of valuable tools such as analgesic dosage tables, sample pain assessment tools, give examples of nondrug interventions, and provide flow charts describing how to treat cancer pain.

The American College of Surgeons (ACoS), along with the Commission on Cancer, report that practice guidelines related to prevention, screening, genetic counseling, early diagnosis, treatment, and follow up care for cancer patients offer a general template for quality and cost-effectiveness. While they do not endorse any specific guidelines, they offer access to guidelines from various well-respected groups and organizations on their web site (http://www.facs.org).

WORLD HEALTH ORGANIZATION

The World Health Organization (WHO) has a program on cancer control that is focused on the prevention, management and monitoring of cancer across the world. They report that their aim is to "develop global strategies to reduce the incidence, morbidity, and mortality of cancer." The WHO encourages and advises countries that belong to the United Nations to develop programs that include prevention, early detection, optimal organization of treatment facilities, and palliative care. They are working with a variety of cancer organizations to explore new initiatives and develop strategies "to reduce cancer suffering, taking into account geographical, epidemiological, cultural, and economic factors." The WHO has developed guidelines for doctors and other health care professionals who treat cancer pain. These guidelines (*Three-Step Analgesic Ladder for Cancer Pain Management*) are widely used for treating cancer pain (see Chapter 4).

NATIONAL COMPREHENSIVE CANCER NETWORK

The National Comprehensive Cancer Network (NCCN) is a nonprofit organization that is an alliance of cancer centers across the country. Physicians and other health care professionals have developed clinical practice guidelines that serve as the practice standard for cancer treatment. Each year a panel of scientific experts updates clinical guidelines, based on advances in medical science and cancer treatment. The American Cancer Society has partnered with NCCN to translate the NCCN *Oncology Practice Guidelines* into a patient-friendly resource. The guidelines offer easy to understand information for patients and family members about treatment options (see Resources).

The *Cancer Pain Treatment Guidelines for Patients* that follow are based on clinical practice guidelines the NCCN developed for oncology specialists. These have been translated into understandable language for the layperson. The guidelines will help you understand your options for pain management. With this information, you'll be better prepared to discuss your choices with your doctor.

The flow charts show step-by-step treatment options for pain control. You'll learn about types of pain and treatment options, important questions to ask your doctor, and information about clinical trials.

Cancer Pain

Treatment Guidelines for Patients

Version I   January 2001

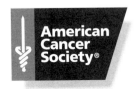

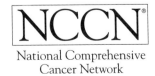

National Comprehensive
Cancer Network

NCCN Clinical Practice Guidelines were developed by a diverse panel of experts. The guidelines are a statement of consensus of its authors regarding the scientific evidence and their views of currently accepted approaches to treatment. The NCCN guidelines are updated as new significant data become available. The Patient Information version will be updated accordingly and will be available on-line through the NCCN and the ACS web sites. To ensure you have the most recent version, you may contact the ACS or the NCCN.

Cancer Pain

Treatment Guidelines for Patients

The mutual goal of the National Comprehensive Cancer Network® (NCCN®) and the American Cancer Society (ACS) partnership is to provide patients and the general public with state-of-the-art cancer treatment information in under-standable language. This information, based on the NCCN's Clinical Practice Guidelines, is intended to assist you in the dialogue with your physician. These guidelines do not replace the expertise and clinical judgment of your physician. Each patient's situation must be evaluated individually. It is important to discuss the guidelines and all information regarding treatment options with your physician. To ensure that you have the most up-to-date version of the guidelines, consult the web sites of the ACS (www.cancer.org) or NCCN (www.nccn.org). You may also call the NCCN at 1-888-909-NCCN or the ACS at 1-800-ACS-2345 for the most recent information.

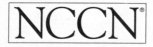

NATIONAL COMPREHENSIVE CANCER NETWORK
MEMBER INSTITUTIONS

CITY OF HOPE CANCER CENTER

DANA-FARBER CANCER INSTITUTE

DUKE COMPRHENSIVE CANCER CENTER

FOX CHASE CANCER CENTER

FRED HUTCHINSON CANCER RESEARCH CENTER

H. LEE MOFFITT CANCER CENTER & RESEARCH INSTITUTE
AT THE UNIVERSITY OF SOUTH FLORIDA

HUNTSMAN CANCER INSTITUTE AT THE UNIVERSITY OF UTAH

ARTHUR G. JAMES CANCER HOSPITAL AND
RICHARD J. SOLOVE RESEARCH INSTITUTE AT THE OHIO STATE UNIVERSITY

JOHNS HOPKINS COMPREHENSIVE CANCER CENTER

MEMORIAL SLOAN-KETTERING CANCER CENTER

ROBERT H. LURIE COMPREHENSIVE CANCER CENTER
OF NORTHWESTERN UNIVERSITY

ROSWELL PARK CANCER INSTITUTE

STANFORD HOSPITAL AND CLINICS

ST. JUDE CHILDREN'S RESEARCH HOSPITAL

UCSF COMPREHENSIVE CANCER CENTER

UNIVERSITY OF TEXAS M. D. ANDERSON CANCER CENTER

UNIVERSITY OF ALABAMA AT BIRMINGHAM
COMPREHENSIVE CANCER CENTER

UNIVERSITY OF MICHIGAN COMPREHENSIVE CANCER CENTER

UNMC/EPPLEY CANCER CENTER
AT THE UNIVERSITY OF NEBRASKA MEDICAL CENTER

This report shows patients how cancer pain is treated at the nation's leading cancer centers. Originally devised for cancer specialists by the National Comprehensive Cancer Network, these treatment guidelines have now been "translated" for the general public by the American Cancer Society. For another copy of these guidelines as well as to learn more information about cancer-related topics, call the American Cancer Society at 1-800-ACS-2345 or the National Comprehensive Cancer Network at 1-888-909-NCCN. Or visit these organizations' web sites at www.cancer.org (ACS) and www.nccn.org (NCCN).

Since 1995, health professionals have looked to the National Comprehensive Cancer Network for guidance on the highest quality, most effective advice on treating cancer. The Network has brought together experts from 19 of the nation's leading cancer centers.

After studying the research results on cancer pain, a panel of these experts has agreed upon specific, state-of-the-art recommendations for treating individuals with cancer-related pain. Every year the panel updates their recommendations based on advances in medical science.

For more than 85 years, the public has turned to the American Cancer Society when they needed information about cancer. The Society's books and brochures have provided comprehensive, current, and understandable information to hundreds of thousands of patients, their families, and friends. This collaboration between the National Comprehensive Cancer Network and the American Cancer Society provides a reliable and understandable source of cancer treatment information for the general public.

Making Decisions About Cancer-Related Pain

About one-third of patients being treated for cancer have pain. More than two-thirds of patients with advanced cancer (cancer that has spread or recurred) have pain. For these patients, controlling pain and managing symptoms are important goals of treatment.

Pain affects all aspects of quality of life. Patients who have chronic pain (pain ranging from mild to severe and present for a long time) may not be able to participate in their regular activities as much, may have sleeping and eating problems, and may be frustrated that family and friends do not always understand how they feel.

Cancer pain is a common problem, but it is one that your cancer care team can treat. Your team may include a social worker, psychologist, oncology nurse, pastor, psychiatrist, medical oncologist, surgeon, and anesthesiologist. The cancer care team will consider each person's medical situation. Remember, each patient is unique and treatment will be developed based on each person's specific pain.

Questions to Ask Your Doctor about Pain Control:

- What can be done to relieve my pain?

- What can we do if the medicine doesn't work?

- What other options do I have for pain control?

- Will the pain medicines have side effects?

- What can be done to manage the side effects?

- Will the treatment limit my activities (i.e., working, driving, etc.)?

To make an informed decision about treatment, patients need to understand the medical terms the doctor uses. This booklet includes background information on cancer pain, explanations of what causes pain, what may prevent effective pain control, and treatments used to treat pain.

What is Pain?

Pain is a sensation that hurts. Normally, pain alerts us to a bodily injury or illness. Everyone feels pain differently so it is important for patients to be able to describe their pain to the doctor or nurse. Patients should explain where the pain is, when it began, how long it lasts, how much it hurts, what it feels like, what makes it better, what makes it worse, and how it affects their life.

TYPES OF PAIN

Acute pain is severe and lasts a relatively short time. It is usually a signal that body tissue is being injured and the pain generally disappears when the injury heals.

Chronic or *persistent pain* may range from mild to severe, and is present to some degree for long periods of time. Some people with chronic pain that is controlled by medicine can have breakthrough pain which is moderate to severe pain that "breaks through" the regular pain medicine given for chronic pain. It is felt for a short time. Breakthrough pain may occur several times a day, even though the proper dose of pain medicine is given for the chronic or persistent pain.

What Causes Pain?

People with cancer may have pain for a variety of reasons. The most common cause of pain in cancer patients is the cancer itself. Pain is caused when cancer spreads into soft tissues (muscle, connective tissue, etc.), organs, or bone; by nerve injury; cancer pressing on a nerve; or increasing pressure in the head. Surgery, radiation therapy, and chemotherapy can also cause pain. This is referred to as treatment-related pain. Patients who have had an arm or leg removed may still be able to feel pain (called *phantom pain*) in the missing limb. This pain is real, but doctors are not sure why it occurs. Several chemotherapy agents cause numbness, tingling, and burning while radiation can cause painful skin irritation.

Sometimes the pain has nothing to do with the cancer or its treatment. Patients with cancer can have headaches, muscle strains, and other aches and pains just like anyone else.

There are three main types of pain: visceral, somatic, and neuropathic.

- Visceral pain involves organs. Pain caused by tissue damage in an organ such as the liver is usually pain that cannot be pinpointed and may be described as throbbing, aching, or sharp.

- Somatic pain involves the bone and is usually in a specific area. It is described as sharp, aching, burning, or throbbing.

- Neuropathic pain is caused by injury to, or compression of, the structures of the peripheral or central nervous system. Nerve injury or compression can be due to an injury of a peripheral nerve, injury to the central nervous system such as the spinal cord, or a combination of injury to both a peripheral nerve and central nervous system.

It is important to know the type of pain present because different pain is treated differently.

What Are the Obstacles to Cancer Pain Relief?

Although most cancer pain can be relieved, controlling cancer patients' pain effectively continues to be a problem. The reasons for this are related to knowledge, beliefs, and fears.

Fear of addiction. Many patients fear that taking opioids (narcotic-like medications), like morphine, will lead to addiction. But this very rarely happens. Just as patients with diabetes have changing needs for insulin, patients with cancer have changing needs for their pain medicines.

Fear of side effects. Patients often take less than the prescribed dose of pain medicines because they are concerned about the side effects that may occur. Most side effects, however, can be prevented or relieved.

Inadequate knowledge. Doctors' and nurses' personal beliefs interfere with adequate management of chronic cancer pain. In the past, doctors and nurses were not well trained to care for patients with chronic pain. They did not always know what medicines were used to control pain. They also were afraid of the possibility that patients would become addicted.

Inadequate pain assessment. Patients often do not mention pain unless asked about it. Some patients believe they must be strong and "tough it out." Patients may not report their pain when they are asked for fear of what the presence of pain may mean. Because they don't mention it, many patients' pain may go unrelieved.

Legal obstacles. When prescribing opioids, especially doses that some might consider high, doctors, pharmacists, and nurses fear actions by drug enforcement agencies. These actions may be exaggerated by professionals and should not be an obstacle to pain relief.

How Will the Doctor Know About the Patient's Pain?

Before starting a plan to manage cancer pain, the doctor needs to know a lot of information about the patient's pain. Collecting this information is called pain assessment or finding out about the patient's pain. This information comes from the patient's physical examination, answers to questions about the patient's medical history, and from family members and friends, especially when the patient is too uncomfortable or too tired to talk.

Patients are asked the following questions about their pain:

- How much does the pain hurt?

- Where is the pain?

- Is the pain

    somatic – such as pain in skin, muscle, or bone described as aching, stabbing, throbbing, or pressure?

    visceral – pain in organs or tissue described as gnawing, cramping, aching, or sharp?

    neuropathic – pain caused by nerve damage described as sharp, tingling, burning, or shooting?

- When did it start?

- How long has it lasted?

- Has the pain changed in any way?

- Is there anything that makes the pain worse or better?

- Is the pain caused by cancer, cancer treatment, or something else?

- Are there any symptoms or side effects from treatment present?

- Do you have a support system available?

- Do you have a history of any mental health problems?

- What do you know or believe about pain and pain control?

After all questions are answered, and the physical examination is done, x-rays and blood tests are done if needed to give more information about the pain. For example if the pain is bone pain and a fracture could be present, an x-ray of the bone is done.

Pain Assessment Tools

Pain assessment tools help patients describe their pain. The pain scale is one tool commonly used to describe the *intensity* of the pain or how much pain the patient is feeling. The pain scales include the numerical rating scale, the visual analog scale, the categorical scale, and the pain faces scale (see figure on page 285).

On the numerical rating scale, the person is asked to identify how much pain they are having by choosing a number from 0 (no pain) to 10 (the worst pain imaginable).

The visual analog scale is a straight line with the left end of the line representing no pain and the right end of the line representing the worst pain. Patients are asked to mark on the line where they think their pain is.

The categorical pain scale has four categories: none, mild, moderate, and severe. Patients are asked to select the category that best describes their pain.

The pain faces scale uses six faces with different expressions on each face. Each face is a person who feels happy because he or she has no pain or feels sad because he or she has some or a lot of pain. The person is asked to choose the face that best describes how he or she is feeling. This rating scale can be used by people age 3 years and older.

Numerical Scale

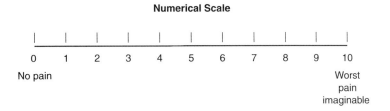

```
|   |   |   |   |   |   |   |   |   |   |
0   1   2   3   4   5   6   7   8   9   10
```

No pain   Worst
                                           pain
                                           imaginable

Visual Analog Scale

No   Worst
pain _____ pain

Directions: Ask the patient to indicate on the line where the pain is in relation to the two extremes. Qualification is only approximate; for example, a midpoint mark would indicate that the pain is approximately half of the worst possible pain.

Categorical Scale

None (0)   Mild (1–3)   Moderate (4–6)   Severe (7–10)

Pain Faces Scale

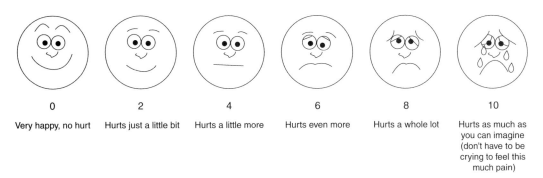

0	2	4	6	8	10
Very happy, no hurt	Hurts just a little bit	Hurts a little more	Hurts even more	Hurts a whole lot	Hurts as much as you can imagine (don't have to be crying to feel this much pain)

Adapted with permission from Whaley L, Wong, D. *Nursing Care of Infants and Children,* ed 3, p. 1070. ©1987 by C.V. Mosby Company. Research reported in Wong D, Baker C. *Pain in children: Comparison of assessment scales. Pediatric Nursing* 14(1):9–17, 1988.

Representative samples of pain intensity rating scales.

How is Cancer Pain Treated?

Once the doctor has assessed the pain, a treatment plan is developed and discussed with the patient. Cancer pain can be treated in several ways, including treating the underlying cancer with chemotherapy, radiation therapy, surgery, or other therapy. Medicines (also called drug therapy) are the main way to treat cancer pain. They include the use of *opioids* (or *narcotics*, the strongest pain relievers available), *non-opioids* (pain relieving medicines that are not opioids, such as acetaminophen and non-steroidal anti-inflammatory drugs, or NSAIDs), and *adjuvant analgesics* (medicines for purposes other than treatment of pain but that help in relieving pain in some situations). Other therapies such as relaxation techniques or biofeedback, physical therapy, anesthesia procedures, and surgical procedures can also be very useful in treating some patients' cancer pain (see pages 288–289).

TREATMENT WITH MEDICINES

Non-opioids. Non-opioids include medicines such as acetaminophen (also called Tylenol®), and NSAIDs such as ibuprofen. These medicines are excellent in relieving bone pain, superficial pain, muscle pain, and some other types of pain. They are the first choice for mild pain. They are also often used with other types of pain medicines to provide greater pain relief.

A maximum daily dose (the amount of medicine taken) is recommended for each of these medicines and taking more can cause significant side effects such as organ damage. Many NSAIDs are now available. They differ in doses, frequency, cost, and to some extent, in their effect and safety.

Side effects will vary, but in general most NSAIDs are associated with gastrointestinal toxicity, with the most serious effects being ulcers and bleeding. They also slow blood clotting, so they must be used cautiously in patients with bleeding or clotting disorders.

Some non-opioids are available without prescription. For others, a prescription is needed. Always follow the doctor's instructions when taking these medicines.

Opioids. Opioids, the strongest pain relieving medicines, are available only by prescription. They include medicines such as codeine, oxycodone, morphine, fentanyl, and hydromorphone, all excellent medicines for the treatment of cancer pain (see chart on page 287).

Opioids are sometimes classified as weak or strong depending on their effectiveness in relieving pain. The weak opioids are used for less severe pain. They often have a non-opioid analgesic (pain-relieving medicine) mixed with them. This mixture limits the dose of the opioid that can be given.

Strong opioids are used for severe pain. Opioids such as morphine, hydromorphone, oxycodone, fentanyl, methadone, and levorphanol may have side effects that can limit the dose of the drug that can be given. Therefore, managing the side effects is critical in effective pain control with any of the opioids. These medicines can be given in a variety of ways.

Opioids are categorized by how quickly they begin to work and how long they are effective. The length of time they are effective is called their duration of action. For example, *sustained-release morphine* (meaning the medicine is released in the body over a longer

Commonly Used Opioids

- Codeine

- Fentanyl

- Hydrocodone

- Hydromorphone

- Levorphanol

- Morphine

- Methadone

- Oxymorphone

- Oxycodone

Weak Opioids: Opioids that can relieve mild to moderate pain, pain with a 4–6 score; usually mixed with other medicines such as acetaminophen or aspirin. Weak opioids include hydrocodone, and codeine. Examples of weak opioids mixed with acetaminophen or aspirin include Tylenol® with codeine, Fiorinal® with codeine, and Phenaphen® with codeine.

Strong Opioids: Opioids that can relieve severe pain, pain with a score of greater than 7; the medicine of choice is morphine; other examples include fentanyl, methadone, levorphanol, hydromorphone, and oxycodone.

period of time) relieves pain for a long time, so a patient takes this medicine less often. *Immediate-release oral morphine* (meaning the medicine is released quickly into the body) is a short-acting opioid, which relieves breakthrough pain quickly. It does not last for long so it is usually used with a long-acting opioid for persistent or chronic pain.

Some opioids such as propoxyphene and meperidine are not recommended for cancer-related pain. Meperidine is *short-acting*, meaning that the dose must be repeated frequently. Its breaks down into another substance which can collect in the body to cause tremors, muscle twitches, and seizures. Propoxyphene can cause serious drug interactions, liver toxicity, tremors, and seizures.

Adjuvant analgesics. Adjuvant analgesics are medicines that have a purpose other than treatment of pain but that help relieve pain in some situations. Adjuvant analgesics used to help relieve cancer pain include the following:

- Antidepressants. Some antidepressants have been found to relieve pain as well as decrease depression. They may relieve neuropathic pain. A prescription is needed for these medicines.

- Anticonvulsants. These medicines are generally used for seizure disorders and are useful in relieving tingling and burning pain, such as neuropathic pain. A prescription is needed for these medicines.

- Steroids. Steroids may be used to relieve pain associated with swelling and with bone pain. A prescription is needed for these medicines.

- Local anesthetics. Local anesthetics can be put on the skin, injected into the spinal canal, and in some cases, be taken by mouth. They are useful for relieving tingling, burning-type pain. A prescription is needed for these medicines.

OTHER TREATMENT METHODS

Surgery. Surgery is used to prevent or control complications of cancer or cancer-related emergencies such as a blockage of the bowel, or compression of vital organs such as the lungs or the spinal cord. Surgery also can be used to reduce the size of the tumor so other treatments will be more effective in treating the cancer.

Radiation Therapy. Radiation therapy is often used to relieve pain caused by cancer that has spread to the bone. The majority of patients with bone metastasis will have significant relief of their pain with radiation therapy.

Chemotherapy. Chemotherapy may be used to reduce the size of a tumor that is causing pain. Hormones also have an important role in controlling some symptoms. For example, in patients with breast or prostate cancer, hormone therapy can reduce the size of a tumor in painful locations such as the bone or soft tissue.

Nerve Blocks. For localized pain that does not respond to other measures or when taking oral medication leads to unacceptable side effects, a local anesthetic, usually combined with a steroid, is injected into a nerve, nerve root, or spinal cord space to block pain. In other selected circumstances, the nerves may be surgically cut to block the pain. In instances when a nerve cannot be blocked, anesthesia can be achieved by injecting opioids into the spinal spaces using a pump to deliver a constant amount of drug.

Non-Medical Therapies. Other non-medical therapies can be effective in relieving pain and improving the patient's ability to function and carry out activities. These therapies include imagery, heat and cold therapy, massage, relaxation, distraction, hypnosis, physical therapy, learning to position for comfort, learning coping skills, and emotional support and counseling.

Imagery involves imagining a pleasant scene, maybe a beach where a person once vacationed or a beautiful mountain retreat. Heat may be applied to areas of pain and for some, cold, such as ice, can be applied to the pain area with good relief. Massage is very relaxing and may relieve muscle spasms and contractions. Relaxation also reduces muscle tension. Distraction involves focusing attention on something other than the pain. Hypnosis is a state of high concentration between sleeping and waking. In a relaxed state, the person is more receptive to suggestion and thus can block the awareness to pain. Transcutaneous electric nerve stimulation (TENS) is a technique that applies a mild electric current to the skin where the pain occurs. The current produces a pleasant sensation and relieves some types of pain. Acupuncture inserts thin needles into the body at points in specific parts of the body to control pain sensations. Physical therapy helps return function and improve mobility. Learning positioning techniques can help relieve pressure on parts of the body and improve circulation. Emotional support and counseling can help relieve anxiety or depression

Patient and Family Education

IMPORTANT MESSAGES FOR THE PATIENT AND FAMILY:

- Your doctor and nurse are concerned about your pain.

- There is no benefit to suffering with pain.

- Pain can usually be well controlled with medicines taken by mouth.

- If these medicines do not work, many other options are available.

- Morphine or morphine-like medicines are often used to relieve pain.

  When these drugs are used to treat cancer pain, addiction is rarely a problem.

  If these medicines are used now, they will still work later.

- Communication with the doctors and nurses is critical.

- Doctors and nurses cannot tell how much pain a patient has unless they are told.

- Doctors and nurses want to know about any problems the pain medicine might be causing, since there are probably ways to make these better.

- The doctor or nurse wants to know if there are any problems getting the medicine or if the patient has concerns about taking them. They have dealt with these issues before and can help.

which can make the pain seem worse. Having pain can also cause people to feel hopeless, helpless, inadequate, and afraid. These feelings, which are normal, can be relieved with counseling and/or medicines. You may discuss these options with your cancer care team and ask for a referral. Information on patient and family education and psychosocial support can be found in the charts on pages 289 and 290, respectively.

It is important for the patient to be able to talk about his or her feelings with someone. This person may be a doctor, nurse, social worker, family or friend, a mental health professional, or other people with cancer. The doctor or nurse will be able to identify mental health professionals with experience in counseling patients with cancer.

What Are the Side Effects of Pain Medicines and How Are They Managed?

The side effects of opioids are easily managed. When first starting to take these medicines, some patients may become drowsy and others may develop some nausea. Vomiting is not common. For most patients, these side effects can be easily managed and usually disappear within 1–3 days. Many different anti-nausea medicines are available today to lessen and control any nausea or vomiting that might occur. To lessen drowsiness, opioids are started at low doses and adjusted or *titrated* (a gradual increase in dose to reach the point of maximum pain relief with the minimum side effects). In older patients, the starting dose is usually lowered.

Psychosocial Support for the Person with Cancer Pain

SUPPORT FOR ADEQUATE PAIN MANAGEMENT

- Psychosocial support is an important part of effective pain control.

- Effective pain control improves the patient's quality of life.

- Pain can be managed by the primary health care team.

- Pharmacy and pharmaceutical companies should be contacted for financial support if payment is a problem for the patient.

- Families may have to speak up and ask for pain management if the patient is not able to.

EMOTIONAL SUPPORT

- Emotional support shows the patient that pain is a problem to be addressed.

- Emotional responses to the pain experience are normal.

- The cancer care team will work with the patient and family to address the pain problem.

- A plan of action will be developed.

- The cancer care team is committed to relieving the patient's pain.

- There is always something else that can be done to try to manage the patient's pain.

SKILLS NEEDED

- Coping skills to control emotional responses, provide pain relief, and enhance a sense of personal control.

- Coping skills for pain emergency such as breathing exercises and distraction techniques.

- Coping skills for chronic pain which includes the above plus relaxation techniques, guided imagery, and hypnosis.

Opioids cause constipation to some degree in most people. Constipation usually occurs after several days of taking opioids and can continue the entire time the medicine is taken. Constipation can be quite painful and may require hospitalization; therefore, it is important to prevent it, if possible. Constipation can be prevented and/or controlled by the following measures:

- Increase intake of liquids,

- Increase dietary fiber, adding such foods as fruits, vegetables, and bran,

- Exercise after getting the doctor's permission,

- Use medicines, such as laxatives and stool softeners, as discussed with the doctor or nurse.

Some people mistakenly think they are allergic to opioids if they become nauseated. Nausea alone usually is not an allergic response. But nausea with a rash or itching may be an allergic reaction. If this occurs, patients should stop taking the medicine and tell their doctor at once. Itching, although rare, may occur at first and can be treated with diphenhydramine (Benadryl®).

Families are often concerned about a slowing of breathing that they associate with a hastening of death. Opioids can slow down breathing but it does not mean that death is near.

Rarely, a patient may experience confusion or "fuzzy thinking", which can be persistent. This can continue to a change in mental function and disorientation, which means that patients do not know where they are or what day of the week it is. The mind wanders and speech is not understandable. These symptoms are called delirium, and the cause of this effect is not clearly understood. It may be necessary to switch to another medicine or reduce the dose of the current drug and add an adjuvant analgesic. Always report any change in mental status to the cancer care team.

MEDICINE TOLERANCE

People who take opioids for pain sometimes find that over time they need to take larger doses. This may be because the pain has increased or because they have developed medicine *tolerance*, also called drug tolerance. Medicine tolerance occurs when the body gets used to the medicine being taken; the medicine does not relieve the pain as well as it once did. Many people do not develop a tolerance to opioids. If tolerance does develop, usually small increases in the dose or a change in the kind of medicine will help relieve the pain. People sometimes confuse tolerance with addiction. The two are very different. Tolerance can occur over time, indicating that the body requires more medicine to achieve the same level of comfort. A need to increase the dose of medicine is not a sign of addiction.

STOPPING AN OPIOID MEDICINE

Stopping opioids suddenly sometimes causes symptoms including a flu-like illness, excessive perspiration, or diarrhea. Opioids are stopped gradually to reduce the chances of any noticeable symptoms occurring. If symptoms do occur, they can be treated and tend to disappear in a few days to a few weeks. The doctor will discuss with the patient the best way to stop taking these medicines.

How Are Pain Medicines Given?

DOSING

Among patients there are enormous differences in the amount (*dose*) of medicine needed to relieve pain, even among patients with similar types of pain. The goal of pain medicine therapy is to provide the maximum benefit to the patient with the least amount of medicine and with the fewest side effects possible. In general, the starting dose will be low, and the amount will be increased until the pain is adequately relieved. This dose adjustment is called titration, that is, adjusting the dose to achieve acceptable pain control. Titration refers to increasing or decreasing the medicine dose. Doctors carefully adjust the doses of pain medicines so there is little possibility of taking too much.

ADMINISTERING MEDICINES

Some people think that if their pain becomes severe, they will need to receive *intramuscular* (IM) injections or "shots." Actually, injections are not commonly used to relieve cancer pain. Giving medicines by mouth (oral administration), is recommended for most patients because it is convenient, well tolerated, and usually is the least expensive. In addition to oral tablets, there are other ways the medicine can be given:

- **Skin patch.** A bandage-like patch placed on the skin, which slowly but continuously releases the medicine through the skin for 2–3 days. One opioid medicine, fentanyl, is available as a skin patch. Giving medicine in this way is less likely to cause nausea and vomiting.

- **Rectal suppositories.** Medicine that dissolves in the rectum and is absorbed by the body.

- **Injections.** Medicines can be given under the skin using a small needle as a *subcutaneous* (SQ) injection; or into the muscle through a needle as an intramuscular (IM) injection, although these are not recommended when repeated injections are needed; as an *intravenous* (IV) injection, or directly into the vein through a needle or thin plastic catheter; as an intrathecal injection, giving medicine directly into the fluid around the spinal cord; or as an epidural injection, giving the medicine into the space between the spinal canal and bones of the back. When the intrathecal or epidural routes are used, opioids may be delivered continuously from a small pump. In situations in which this method will be used over a long period of time, the pump can be placed under the skin.

- **Patient-controlled analgesia (PCA).** When pain relief is needed, the patient can receive a preset dose of pain medicine by pressing a button on a computerized pump that is connected to a small tube in the body. The medicine is injected into the vein (intravenously), just under the skin (subcutaneously), or into the spinal area.

The way the medicine is given is influenced by several factors, such as patients having difficulty taking pills, the presence of irritating side effects, or pain that is not controlled with an opioid given by mouth. Patients who are having difficulty taking their medicines should ask their doctor about a different method of administration.

SCHEDULING

When the pain occurs day after day, medicines are given on an around-the-clock (ATC) schedule to ensure that the body always has a supply. In the past, medicines were given only on an as needed basis, or PRN, with the patient waiting until they were in pain. This type of schedule allowed periods of severe pain. Around-the-clock dosing is preferred. This means giving the medicine on a regular basis, whether the patient is in pain or not. In some situations patients are instructed to take a pain medicine as needed. This is usually along with an ATC medicine that they are already taking.

Are There Clinical Trials Studying New Pain Treatments?

All drugs used to treat pain, cancer, or other diseases must undergo clinical trials in order to determine their safety and effectiveness before the Food and Drug Administration (FDA) can approve them for use.

When studying promising new or experimental treatments, researchers want to know:

- Does this new type of treatment work better than other treatments already available?

- What side effects does the treatment cause?

- Do the benefits outweigh the risks, including side effects?

- Which patients will the treatment most likely help?

During cancer treatment, the doctor may suggest taking part in a clinical trial of a new treatment for pain. Scientists conduct clinical trials only when they believe that the treatment being studied may be better than other treatments.

The purpose of the study is to find out if the new treatment will work better than the standard treatment and if the side effects are worse or less. The new therapy may have some side effects, which the doctor will discuss with the patient before the clinical trial is started.

Taking part in any clinical trial is completely voluntary. Doctors and nurses explain the study in detail and provide a consent form to read and sign. This form states that the patient understands the risks and wants to participate. Even after signing the form and the trial begins, the patient may leave the study at any time, for any reason.

Taking part in the study will not keep anyone from getting other medical care they may need. Patients should always check with their health insurance company to find out whether it will cover the costs of taking part in a clinical trial.

Participating in a clinical trial evaluating new, improved methods for managing cancer pain may help the patient directly, and it may help other people with cancer pain in the future. For these reasons, members of the National Comprehensive Cancer Network and the American Cancer Society encourage participation in clinical trials.

Assessment and Treatment Guidelines

'Decision Trees'

The "decision trees", or algorithms, on the following pages represent decisions about treatment of cancer pain based on how bad the pain is. Each tree shows step-by-step how you and your doctor can make treatment choices.

Keep in mind, this information is not meant to be used without the expertise of your own doctor who is familiar with your situation, medical history, and personal preferences.

The NCCN guidelines are updated as new significant data become available. To ensure you have the most recent version, consult the web sites of the ACS (www.cancer.org) or NCCN (www.nccn.org). You may also call the NCCN at 1-888-909-NCCN or the ACS at 1-800-ACS-2345 for the most recent information on these guidelines or on cancer in general.

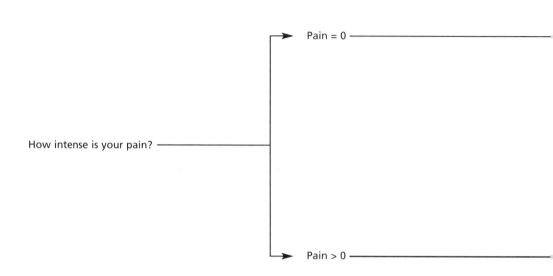

How intense is your pain? ——————————

Pain = 0 ——————————————

Pain > 0 ——————————————

ASSESSING THE PATIENT'S PAIN (DOES THE PATIENT HAVE PAIN?)

Since all patients can have cancer pain but not all patients do, the first step in making a decision about treatment is to find out if the patient is having pain. The patient is asked to rate their pain using a visual rating scale of 1–10 (see numerical scale on page 285). A score of 0 indicates that no pain is present and a rat-

Decision Tree for Assessment of Cancer-Related Pain

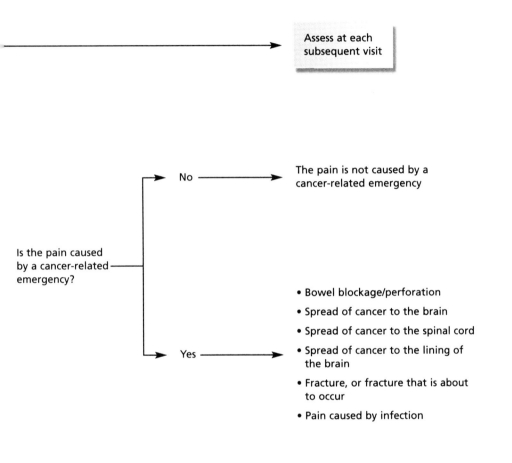

Assess at each subsequent visit

No ──→ The pain is not caused by a cancer-related emergency

Is the pain caused by a cancer-related emergency?

Yes ──→
- Bowel blockage/perforation
- Spread of cancer to the brain
- Spread of cancer to the spinal cord
- Spread of cancer to the lining of the brain
- Fracture, or fracture that is about to occur
- Pain caused by infection

ing of 10 indicates the pain is the worst it can be. If the patient has no pain, he or she will be asked about it on each subsequent visit to the doctor. If the patient is in pain, the doctor will do a thorough assessment, or evaluation, so appropriate treatment can be planned.

The immediate goal of the first pain assessment is to find out if the pain is present because of a medical emergency. If one is present, it will require immediate treatment. Because tumors can invade bone, nerves, and tissue, there are several cancer pain emergencies that must be treated quickly. These include:

- a fracture (break in a bone) or near fracture of a bone that is able to carry weight, such as a vertebra in the back or the hip bone;

- a bowel blockage or perforation (hole in the wall of the bowel) caused by tumor growth;

NOTES

- metastasis, or spread of the cancer to the brain, spinal cord, or the lining of the brain; and

- pain caused by an infection in just one part of the body, or one that involves the entire body (septicemia).

The patient will be asked several questions about their pain. (see *How Will The Doctor Know About The Patient's Pain?* on pages 283 and 284). The patient's completed numerical rating scale will help the doctor understand how intense, or bad, the pain is.

NOTES

_____

_____

_____

_____

_____

_____

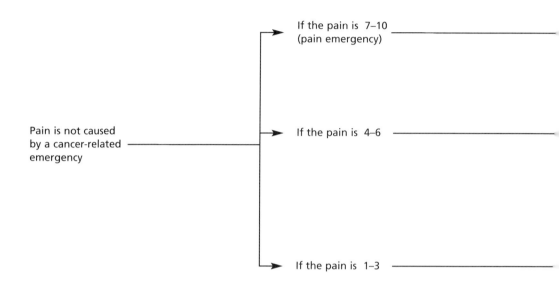

If the pain is 7–10
(pain emergency) _____

Pain is not caused
by a cancer-related ———
emergency

If the pain is 4–6 _____

If the pain is 1–3 _____

Pain is caused by a
cancer-related emergency _____

Keep in mind this information is not meant to be used without the expertise of your own physician who is familiar with your situation, medical history, and personal preferences.

INITIAL TREATMENT

Once the assessment is completed, the pain treatment is planned. Treatment options will be discussed with the patient. If it is a pain emergency, the cause of the pain will be treated. If no emergency situation is present, and the patient's pain is greater than 7 on the visual pain scale, the patient will be given a short-acting opioid and the dose will be increased rapidly. A bowel program will be started to lower the chances of constipation. A medicine may be given to prevent nausea and vomiting, a side effect from the opioid. During this time

Decision Tree for Initial Treatment of Cancer-Related Pain

INITIAL TREATMENT

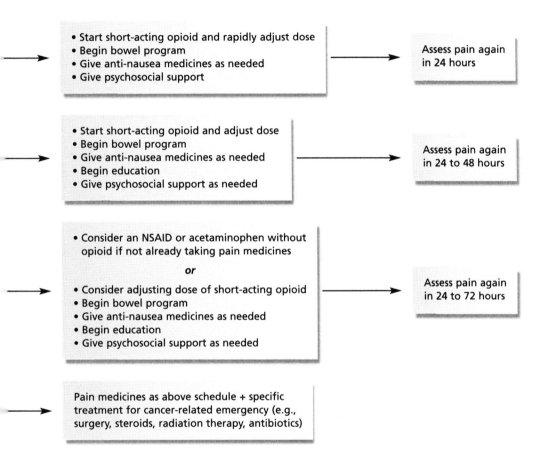

- Start short-acting opioid and rapidly adjust dose
- Begin bowel program
- Give anti-nausea medicines as needed
- Give psychosocial support

→ Assess pain again in 24 hours

- Start short-acting opioid and adjust dose
- Begin bowel program
- Give anti-nausea medicines as needed
- Begin education
- Give psychosocial support as needed

→ Assess pain again in 24 to 48 hours

- Consider an NSAID or acetaminophen without opioid if not already taking pain medicines

or

- Consider adjusting dose of short-acting opioid
- Begin bowel program
- Give anti-nausea medicines as needed
- Begin education
- Give psychosocial support as needed

→ Assess pain again in 24 to 72 hours

Pain medicines as above schedule + specific treatment for cancer-related emergency (e.g., surgery, steroids, radiation therapy, antibiotics)

the patient will need the support of the cancer care team, family, and friends (refer to *Psychosocial Support for the Person with Cancer Pain* on page 290). In about 24 hours the pain will be reevaluated using the pain rating scale.

If the pain is rated from 4 to 6, a short-acting opioid will be given with dose titrated, or

adjusted (either increased or decreased) until the pain is relieved. The bowel preparation and "as needed" anti-nausea medicines will be started. Pain will be reassessed, or re-evaluated, in about 24 to 48 hours by the doctor or nurse.

If the pain is rated from 1 to 3, an NSAID or a short-acting opioid is an option. A bowel regimen will be started and anti-nausea medicines will be given "as needed". An education program should be started to establish a common language for talking about pain with the health care team (refer to *Patient and Family Education* on page 289). One goal of the education program is to understand why patients do not always get effective pain control and to make sure patients have the information they need to follow the prescribed plan. Beliefs that create the greatest problems for patients in taking their pain medicines are fear of addiction, concerns about side effects, concerns about tolerance, and the need to be stoic. Patients also should know what medicines they should stop taking and when to call the doctor.

NOTES

Pain that is caused by a cancer-related emergency will be treated with analgesics, or pain medicines, according to the above treatment plan. Specific treatment will also be given for the emergency (for example, surgery, radiation therapy, antibiotics, or steroids).

In about 24 to 72 hours after the pain treatment is begun, the patient will complete another visual pain scale. Further changes in the pain treatment will be made based on how well the patient's pain is being controlled with the pain medicine.

NOTES

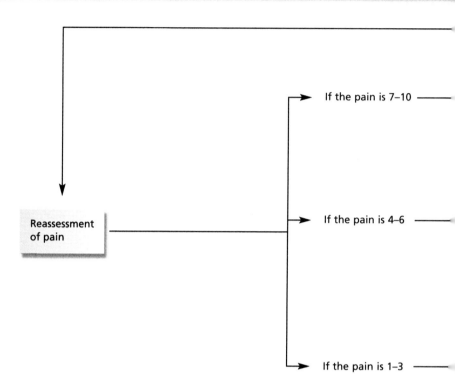

If the pain is 7–10 ——

Reassessment of pain — If the pain is 4–6 ——

If the pain is 1–3 ——

Keep in mind this information is not meant to be used without the expertise of your own physician who is familiar with your situation, medical history, and personal preferences.

SUBSEQUENT TREATMENT

A score of 7 to 10 means that the pain is not better or it has gotten worse. Since the goal of pain treatment is to reach a lower score on the pain scale, the doctor will reconsider the original cause of pain. This means that the doctor will look once again at the medical history and consider if the original cause of pain is still causing the current pain.

Next, the patient's pain medicine dose will be adjusted. For example, more of the medicine may be given or a different medicine may be given. Additional treatments for specific types of pain may be added to the current pain medicines. For example, NSAIDs might be added with bone pain or pain with inflammation. Anti-depressants might be added for burning neuropathic pain. Non-medical therapies will also be considered (see pages 288–289). The pain will be re-evaluated in about 24 hours.

If the patient's pain score is 4 to 6, the doctor will continue to adjust the medicine dose. Other treatments (as mentioned above) may also be added. After changes have been made in the pain treatment plan, the patient's pain will be

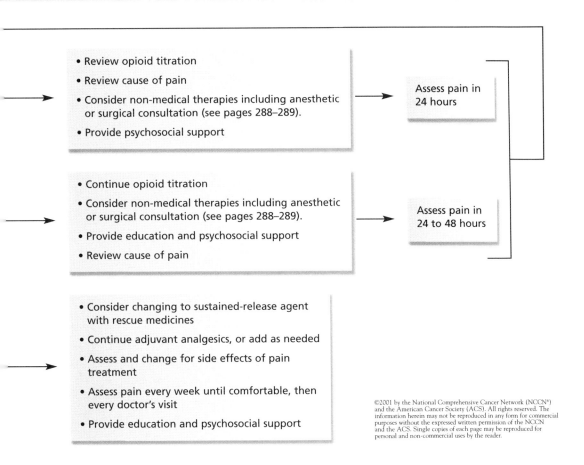

- Review opioid titration
- Review cause of pain
- Consider non-medical therapies including anesthetic or surgical consultation (see pages 288–289).
- Provide psychosocial support

Assess pain in 24 hours

- Continue opioid titration
- Consider non-medical therapies including anesthetic or surgical consultation (see pages 288–289).
- Provide education and psychosocial support
- Review cause of pain

Assess pain in 24 to 48 hours

- Consider changing to sustained-release agent with rescue medicines
- Continue adjuvant analgesics, or add as needed
- Assess and change for side effects of pain treatment
- Assess pain every week until comfortable, then every doctor's visit
- Provide education and psychosocial support

assessed in about 24 to 48 hours to see if it is any better.

If the pain is rated 3 or less, the pain medicine may be switched to a sustained-released oral medicine, which means the patient can take the medicine less often. Medicine will be given if the patient has breakthrough pain. Other medicines that have been added to the pain treatment plan will be continued if they are still needed for the pain. Education and support will be continued as needed. The side effects of pain medicines will be considered and medicines will be changed if needed to reduce side effects. Pain will be assessed every week until the patient is comfortable, then with every visit to the doctor.

The goal of pain treatment is to continue to reduce the amount of pain the patient has to a level less than 4. Pain is assessed after each change in treatment. Patient and family education and psychosocial support, important components of cancer pain treatment, are continued throughout treatment. After each pain assessment, pain treatment will be adjusted based on the intensity of the pain using the pain scale.

NOTES

The Cancer Pain Treatment Guidelines for Patients were developed by a diverse group of experts and were based on the NCCN clinical practice guidelines. These patient guidelines were translated, reviewed, and published with help from the following individuals.

Terri Ades, MS, RN, CS, AOCN
American Cancer Society
Health Content Products

Matthew J. Loscalzo, MSW
Johns Hopkins Oncology Center

Cameron Muir, MD
Robert H. Lurie
Comprehensive Cancer Center
of Northwestern University

Susan Shinagawa
Patient Representative

Dia Taylor
National Comprehensive
Cancer Network

Sharon M. Weinstein, MD
Huntsman Cancer Institute
at the University of Utah

Rodger Winn, MD
National Comprehensive
Cancer Network

The original NCCN Cancer Pain Treatment Guidelines were developed by the following NCCN Panel Members.

Costantino Benedetti, MD
Arthur G. James Cancer Hospital
& Richard J. Solove Research
Institute at Ohio State University

Charles Brock, MD
H. Lee Moffitt Cancer Center
and Research Institute at the
University of South Florida

Charles Cleeland, PhD
University of Texas
M. D. Anderson Cancer Center

Nessa Coyle, RN
Memorial Sloan-Kettering
Cancer Center

James E. Dube', PharmD
UNMC/Eppley Cancer Center
at the University of Nebraska
Medical Center

Betty Ferrell, PhD
City of Hope National
Medical Center

Stuart A. Grossman, MD / Chair
Johns Hopkins Oncology Center

Samuel Hassenbusch III, MD, PhD
University of Texas
M. D. Anderson Cancer Center

Nora A. Janjan, MD
University of Texas
M. D. Anderson Cancer Center

Mark J. Lema, MD, PhD
Roswell Park Cancer Institute

Michael H. Levy, MD, PhD
Fox Chase Cancer Center

Matthew J. Loscalzo, MSW
Johns Hopkins Oncology Center

Maureen Lynch, RN, NP
Dana-Farber Cancer Institute

Cameron Muir, MD
Robert H. Lurie
Comprehensive Cancer Center
of Northwestern University

Linda Oakes, RN
St. Jude Children's
Research Hospital

Alison M. O'Neill, MD
University of Alabama
at Birmingham
Comprehensive Cancer Center

Richard Payne, MD
Memorial Sloan-Kettering
Cancer Center

Karen L. Syrjala, PhD
Fred Hutchinson
Cancer Research Center

Susan Urba, MD
University of Michigan
Comprehensive Cancer Center

Sharon M. Weinstein, MD
Huntsman Cancer Institute
at the University of Utah

Resources

Listings in this section represent organizations that operate on a national level and provide some type of service or resource to consumers related to cancer pain. This list is designed to give you a starting point for seeking information, support, and needed resources. If you have a question that cannot be answered by one of the sources listed here, do not give up. Many of these organizations provide referrals, and your questions may be directed to other organizations or individuals.

Most of the organizations listed can be contacted via phone, fax, or e-mail, and some through their web site. Many of the web sites provide much of the same information that is available by mail. Some organizations are solely web-based and will require Internet access. Keep in mind that new web sites appear daily while old ones expand, move, or disappear entirely. Some of the web sites given below, or their content, may be different by the time you read this book. Often, a simple Internet search will point you to the new web site for a given organization.

AMERICAN CANCER SOCIETY RESOURCES AND PROGRAMS

The American Cancer Society (ACS) provides educational materials and information on cancer, maintains several patient programs, and directs people to services in their community. To find your local office, contact the Division office for your state or region, call 800-ACS-2345, or visit our web site (*http://www.cancer.or*g).

Cancer Survivors Network

American Cancer Society
1599 Clifton Road, NE
Atlanta, GA 30329-4251
Toll-Free: 800-ACS-2345
Web site: *http://www.acscsn.org*

This network provides an on-line community that welcomes cancer survivors, friends, and families to share and communicate with others with similar interests and experiences. The program offers a vibrant community of real people supporting one another and sharing personal experiences with cancer. The web site enables registered members to have live, private chats, to create personal web pages to share experiences, thoughts, and wisdom, to help people create personal support communities of people who share common concerns and interests, and offers information about resources.

I Can Cope

American Cancer Society
1599 Clifton Road, NE
Atlanta, GA 30329-4251
Toll-Free: 800-ACS-2345
Web site: *http://www.cancer.org*

This program addresses the educational and psychological needs of people with cancer and their families. A series of eight classes discusses the disease, coping with daily health problems, controlling cancer-related pain, nutrition for the person with cancer, expressing feelings, living with limitations, and local resources. Through lectures, group discussions, and study assignments, the course helps people with cancer regain a sense of control over their lives.

Man to Man

American Cancer Society
1599 Clifton Road, NE
Atlanta, GA 30329-4251
Toll-Free: 800-ACS-2345
Web site: *http://www.cancer.org*

This program provides accurate, factual information to men and their partners about prostate cancer in a supportive environment following essential guidelines that assure program integrity and credibility. Man to Man is an ideal vehicle by which new relationships are formed between patients/survivors and care providers with a two-way exchange of information, trust, and respect.

Reach to Recovery

American Cancer Society
1599 Clifton Road, NE
Atlanta, GA 30329-4251
Toll-Free: 800-ACS-2345
Web site: *http://www.cancer.org*

This program is designed to help patients with breast cancer cope with their diagnosis, treatment, and recovery. The volunteers for this program are women who have had breast cancer and are specially trained to share their knowledge and experiences in a supportive and nonintrusive manner. Ongoing support groups are available to help women deal with the challenges of breast cancer. Reach to Recovery also provides early support to women who may have breast cancer or have just been diagnosed with cancer.

PAIN AND CANCER INFORMATION

The organizations listed below provide information about several different types of cancer and the pain associated with cancer. Most of the web sites provided are searchable under the topic of pain and some have special sections devoted exclusively to pain and related issues. The agencies, organizations, corporations, and publications represented in this resource guide are not necessarily endorsed by the American Cancer Society. This guide is provided for assistance in obtaining information only.

AMC Cancer Research Center & Foundation

1600 Pierce Street
Denver, CO 80214
Toll-Free: 800-525-3777
Phone: 303-239-3422
Fax: 303-233-1863
Web site: *http://www.amc.org*

The AMC Cancer Research Center and Foundation is a nonprofit research institute dedicated to the prevention of cancer and other chronic diseases. The Center offers the Cancer Information and Counseling Line (CICL), a toll-free line staffed by professionals with degrees in counseling or related health areas. The CICL provides information and materials on cancer as well as counseling and support referrals to local community and medical support. CICL services are available for patients, families, survivors, and the public. The web site contains general information about breast, colorectal, and prostate cancer and the pain associated with cancer, as well as information on nutrition, exercise, sun safety, and smoking information, and links to cancer-related resources.

American Medical Association (AMA)

515 North State Street

Chicago, IL 60610

Toll-Free: 800-262-3211

Phone: 312-464-5000

Fax: 312-464-5600

Web site: *http://www.ama-assn.org*

The AMA develops and promotes standards in medical practice, research, and education. Under the consumer health information section, the web site contains databases on physicians and hospitals, which can be searched by medical specialty. A pull-down menu of specific conditions is also provided.

American Society for Therapeutic Radiology and Oncology (ASTRO)

12500 Fair Lakes Circle, Suite 375

Fairfax, VA 22033-3882

Toll-Free: 800-962-7876

Phone: 703-502-1550

Fax: 703-502-7852

Web site: *http://www.astro.org*

Focusing on the use of radiation therapy for the treatment of cancer, this society's web site includes an overview of radiation therapy and a list of frequently asked questions.

American Society of Clinical Oncology (ASCO)

225 Reinekers Lane, Suite 650

Alexandria, VA 22314

Toll-Free: 888-651-3038

Phone: 703-299-0150

Fax: 703-299-1044

Web site: *http://www.asco.org*

ASCO is an international medical society representing about 10,000 cancer specialists involved in clinical research and patient care. The ASCO web site is a resource for cancer patients, doctors, and researchers and includes patient guides, a glossary of cancer terms, an ASCO member oncologist locator, news and information about different cancers and drug treatments, information about cancer legislation, summaries of government reports, and links to related sites.

Association of Community Cancer Centers (ACCC)

11600 Nebel Street, Suite 201

Rockville, MD 20852-2557

Phone: 301-984-9496

Fax: 301-770-1949

Web site: *http://www.accc-cancer.org*

This national organization includes over 600 medical centers, hospitals, and cancer programs. This web site contains a searchable database of cancer centers listed by state as well as information about oncology drugs (registration is required), and specific cancers.

Cancer Research Institute (CRI)

681 Fifth Avenue

New York, NY 10022

Toll-Free: 800-99-CANCER

Phone: 212-688-7515

Fax: 212-832-9376

Web site: *http://www.cancerresearch.org*

An institute funding cancer research and providing public information on cancer immunology and cancer treatment, the CRI helps locate immunotherapy clinical trials, and offers a cancer reference guide and other informational booklets.

Centers for Disease Control and Prevention (CDC)

1600 Clifton Road, NE

Atlanta, GA 30333

Toll-Free: 888-842-6355

Phone: 404-639-3534

Web site: *http://www.cdc.gov/cancer*

The CDC is an agency of the United States Department of Health and Human Services. Their mission is to promote health and quality of life by preventing and controlling disease, injury, and disability. The CDC provides information about chronic diseases, such as cancer. *Spanish-speaking staff and Spanish materials are available.*

City of Hope Pain/Palliative Care Resource Center

1500 East Duarte Road
Duarte, CA 91010
Phone: 626-359-8111, ext. 63829
Fax: 626-301-8941
Web site: *http://prc.coh.org*

The City of Hope Pain/Palliative Care Resource Center serves as a clearinghouse to disseminate information and resources to assist health professionals with improving the quality of pain management. They offer information on a variety of topics including pain assessment tools, patient education materials, quality assurance materials, research instruments, and end of life resources. The web site provides a list of publications and other materials available for order. Some publications are available on-line. *Some Spanish materials are available.*

Mayo Clinic

Web site: *http://www.mayoclinic.com*

This web site contains a database searchable by health conditions. It also offers questions and answers from specialists at the Mayo Clinic, as well as healthy lifestyle planners.

Medscape

Web site: *http://www.medscape.com*

Although registration is required to view some of the content, this web site offers a great deal of information on prescription drugs as well as medical articles. There are also links to several organizations, cancer centers, database and education web sites, journals, and government sites. The web site is also searchable by key word. Registration is free.

National Cancer Institute (NCI)

NCI Public Inquiries Office
Building 31, Room 10A03
31 Center Drive, MSC 2580
Bethesda, MD 20892-2580
Toll-Free: 800-4-CANCER
Web site: *http://www.cancer.gov*

This government agency provides cancer information through several services (see list below). *Spanish-speaking staff and Spanish materials are available.*

CANCERLIT (Bibliographic Database)

Web site: *http://cnetdb.nci.nih.gov/cancerlit.html*

This searchable site is maintained by the NCI and contains cancer and pain articles published in medical and scientific journals, books, government reports, and articles that were presented at national meetings. A link to the PDQ (CancerNet/NCI database) search engine is provided which allows you to search for clinical trials by state, city, and type of cancer.

CancerTrials

Web site: *http://cancertrials.nci.nih.gov*

Maintained by the NCI, this site offers information about on-going cancer clinical trials and explanations of what a trial is and what is involved. A link to the PDQ (CancerNet/NCI database) search engine is provided which allows you to search for clinical trials by state, city, and type of cancer. This site also offers the *Clinical Trials and Insurance Coverage: A Resource Guide* at *http:/cancertrials.nci.nih.gov/understanding/indepth/insurance/index.html.* The guide offers information regarding the cost of clinical trials and how to determine if you will be covered under your health plan. Information about financial assistance programs for the needy is also available.

CancerFax

Fax: 301-402-5874

CancerFax includes information about cancer treatment, screening, prevention, and supportive care. To obtain a contents list, dial the fax number from a fax machine hand set and follow the recorded instructions.

CancerNet

Web site: *http://cancernet.gov*

Web site (Spanish version): *http://cancernet.gov/sp_menu.htm*

Web site (On-line ordering): *http://publications.nci.nih.gov*

A comprehensive web site that contains information on diagnosis, treatment, support, resources, literature, clinical trials, prevention and risk factors, and testing.

Up to 20 publications can be ordered on-line. The publications list is searchable. *Some publications are available in Spanish.*

Cancer Information Service (CIS)

Toll-Free: 800-4-CANCER

Web site: *http://cis.nci.nih.gov*

The CIS provides information to consumers and health care professionals. Call CIS for a referral to a pain control clinic or support group in your area. The web site contains a wealth of information including pamphlets and brochures on cancer diagnosis, treatment, research, and prevention. *Spanish-speaking staff are available.*

National Center for Complementary and Alternative Medicine (NCCAM)

Web site: *http://altmed.od.nih.gov*

This NIH web site provides information on some complementary and alternative methods being promoted to treat different diseases.

National Comprehensive Cancer Network (NCCN)

50 Huntingdon Pike, Suite 200

Rockledge, PA 19046

Toll-Free: 800-909-NCCN

Phone: 215-728-4788

Fax: 215-728-3877

Web site: *http://www.nccn.org*

The NCCN is a nonprofit organization that is an alliance of cancer centers. The American Cancer Society has partnered with NCCN to translate the NCCN Clinical Practice Guidelines into a patient-friendly resource. The guidelines offer easy to understand information for patients and family members about treatment options for each stage of cancer. The treatment guidelines for patients are available for breast, prostate, and colon and rectal cancer, as well as for nausea and vomiting and cancer pain. More guidelines are currently being developed. Call ACS for the latest guidelines or view them online at either www.cancer.org or www.nccn.org.

National Library of Medicine (includes MEDLINE)

Web site: *http://www.nlm.nih.gov*

This National Institutes of Health web site provides a search engine for health, medical, and scientific literature and research as well as links to other government resources.

PubMed

Web site: *http://www.ncbi.nlm.nih.gov/PubMed*

As part of the National Library of Medicine (NLM), this web site provides access to literature references in Medline and other databases, with links to on-line journals. The site is searchable by key word.

NLM Gateway

Web site: *http://gateway.nlm.nih.gov/gw/Cmd*

This site offers links to searchable databases and allows users to search simultaneously in multiple retrieval systems at the NLM.

OncoLink

University of Pennsylvania Cancer Center

Web site: *http://www.oncolink.com*

This web site provides information on cancer including clinical trials, support groups, educational materials, cancer screening and prevention, financial questions, and other resources for people with cancer.

PATIENT AND FAMILY SERVICES

American Association of Retired People (AARP)

Dept. # 258390

P.O. Box 40011

Roanoke, VA 24022

Toll-Free: 800-456-2277

Web site: *http://www.aarp.org*

Web site (for Pharmacy Service): *http://www.rpspharmacy.com*

The AARP is a nonprofit membership organization with a commitment to older adults. It provides a variety of services to its members including information on managed care, Medicare, Medicaid, long-term care, and other issues of interest. Membership is open to anyone 50 years old or older. The web site includes information on a member pharmacy service that offers discounts on drugs used for cancer treatment and pain relief.

Cancer Care, Inc.

275 Seventh Avenue
New York, NY 10001
Toll-Free (Counseling): 800-813-HOPE
Phone: 212- 302-2400
Fax: 212- 719-0263
Web site: *http://www.cancercare.org*
Web site (Spanish version): *http://www.cancercare.org/spanishmenu.htm*

A nonprofit social service agency, Cancer Care, Inc. provides counseling and guidance to help people with cancer, their families, and friends cope with the impact of cancer. The web site includes detailed information on specific cancers and cancer treatment, cancer pain, clinical trials, and links to other sites. The organization also provides videos, support groups (online, telephone, and face-to-face), workshops, seminars and clinics, a newsletter, and other publications to interested consumers. *Spanish-speaking staff are available.*

Candlelighters Childhood Cancer Foundation (CCCF)

3910 Warner Street
Kensington, MD 20895
Toll-Free: 800-366-2223
Phone: 301-962-3520
Fax: 301-962-3521
Web site: *http://www.candlelighters.org*

Candlelighters is an international, nonprofit organization whose mission is to educate, support, serve, and advocate for families of children with cancer, survivors of childhood cancer, and the health care professionals who care for them. CCCF provides a network of parent support groups, an Ombudsman Program offering legal assistance to families of children with cancer and adult survivors of childhood cancer, and publications.

Encore Plus Programs of the YWCA

Office of Women's Health Advocacy
624 Ninth Street, NW, Third Floor
Washington, DC 20001-5303
Toll-Free: 800-953-7587
Phone: 202-467-0801 or 202-626-0700
Fax: 202-783-7123
Web site: *http://www.ywca.org*

Sponsored by the YWCA, this community-based program provides support to women undergoing breast cancer treatment including exercise programs. Charges for the program vary by location.

Health Insurance Association of America

555 13th Street, NW, Suite 600 East
Washington, DC 20004
Toll-Free: 800-879-4422
Phone: 202-824-1600
Fax: 202-824-1722
Web site: *http://www.hiaa.org*

This association represents most United States health insurance companies. The web site contains insurance guides and general insurance information, and an annual directory and survey of hospitals, along with other information.

Leukemia and Lymphoma Society

1311 Mamaroneck Avenue
Third Floor
White Plains, NY 10605
Toll-Free: 800-955-4572
Phone: 914-949-5213
Fax: 914-949-6691
Web site: *http://www.leukemia.org*

The Leukemia and Lymphoma Society is a national voluntary health agency dedicated to curing leukemia, lymphoma, Hodgkin's disease, and myeloma, and improving the quality of life of patients and their families. This organization was formerly known as the Leukemia Society of America (LSA). Patient service programs and resources include financial assistance for select approved drugs related to treatment and/or control of leukemia, lymphoma, Hodgkin's disease, and myeloma; other treatment-related expenses; and for transportation to and from a doctor's office, hospital, treatment center, or support group, First Connection, a telephone-based peer support network for newly diagnosed patients and family members, patient education and information referral to local community resources and local chapters, and support groups.

Medicare Hotline

Department of Health and Human Services
Toll-Free: 800-MEDICAR
Toll-Free Info Line: 800-633-4227
Web site: *http://www.medicare.gov*
Web site: *http://www.ssa.gov*

Call the toll-free number to receive information about local services and Medicare benefits. The web site may be difficult to access.

National Bone Marrow Transplant Link (NBMT Link)

20411 West 12 Mile Road, Suite 108
Southfield, MI 48076
Toll-Free: 800-546-5268
Phone: 248-358-1886
Fax: 248-932-8483
Web site: *http://www.comnet.org/nbmtlink*

This organization serves as an information center for prospective Bone Marrow Transplant (BMT) patients as well as a resource for health professionals. NBMT Link provides peer support to BMT patients and their families over the telephone. The peer-support volunteers are BMT transplant survivors who have been specially trained. The NBMT Link web site also offers NBMT's publications and answers to frequently asked questions.

National Coalition for Cancer Survivorship (NCCS)

1010 Wayne Avenue
Silver Spring, MD 20910
Toll-Free: 888-937-6227

Phone: 301-650-8868 or 301-565-8195 (For publications)

Fax: 301-565-9670

Web site: *http://www.cansearch.org*

Web site (Spanish version): *http://www.cansearch.org/spanish/index.html*

The NCCS is a network of independent organizations working in the area of cancer survivorship and support. The web site offers links to on-line cancer resources, support groups, survivorship programs, and a newsletter.

National Family Caregivers Association (NFCA)

10400 Connecticut Avenue, Suite 500

Kensington, MD 20895-3944

Toll-Free: 800-896-3650

Phone: 301-942-6430

Fax: 301-942-2302

Web site: *http://www.nfcacares.org*

This organization is a national, nonprofit, membership association whose mission is to promote caregiving through education, support, public awareness, and advocacy. The NFCA provides referrals to national resources for caregivers and offers a bereavement kit for caregivers for a fee. The NFCA web site provides a report on the status of family caregivers and ten tips for family caregivers.

National Lymphedema Network (NLN)

Latham Square

1611 Telegraph Avenue, Suite 1111

Oakland, CA 94612-2138

Toll-Free (Hotline): 800-541-3259

Phone: 510-208-3200

Fax: 510-208-3110

Web site: *http://www.lymphnet.org*

The web site for this nonprofit agency offers information and education about lymphedema, a referral service to medical and therapeutic treatment centers, and information on locating or establishing local support groups. It publishes a newsletter, which contains articles on lymphedema and related topics, including a resource guide of treatment centers, physicians, therapists, and suppliers. The NLN lists over 100 support groups.

National Self-Help Clearinghouse

Graduate School and University Center of the City University of New York

365 Fifth Avenue, Suite 3300

New York, NY 10016

Phone: 212-817-1822

Fax: 212-817-2990

Web site: *http://www.selfhelpweb.org*

A nonprofit organization that provides access to regional self-help services.

National Viatical Association

1030 15th Street, Suite 870

Washington, DC 20005

Phone: 202-347-7361

Toll-Free: 800-741-9465

Fax: 202-393-0336

Web site: *http://nationalviatical.org*

This organization provides information on the pre-death purchase of life insurance policies. The web site offers information on member organizations, the latest news in the industry, and information on the ethics behind this kind of transaction.

Pharmaceutical Research and Manufacturers Association of America (PhRMA)

1100 15th Street, NW, Suite 900

Washington, DC 20005

Phone: 202-835-3400

Fax: 202-835-3414

Web site: *http://www.phrma.org*

PhRMA provides information about member pharmaceutical companies and drugs that are currently available, in clinical trials, or under development. The web site includes a directory of patient assistance programs for prescription drugs and a database of new medications for cancer and other diseases.

Social Security Administration

Department of Health and Human Services

Toll-Free: 800-772-1213

Web site: *http://www.ssa.gov*

Call the toll-free number to receive information about local services.

TRICARE (formerly CHAMPUS)

Web site: *http://www.tricare.osd.mil*

TRICARE is part of the military health care system. The web site offers a link to TRICARE regional offices and a list of phone numbers.

Viatical Association of America

1200 19th Street, NW

Washington, DC 20036-2412

Phone: 202-429-5129

Fax: 202-429-5113

Web site: *http://www.viatical.org*

A tax-exempt trade association composed of viatical settlement brokers and funding companies. The web site offers contact information on the over 30 member companies belonging to the association and information on viatical settlements.

US TOO International

930 N. York Road, Suite 50

Hinsdale, IL 60521

Toll-Free: 800-808-7866

Phone: 630-323-1002

Fax: 630-323-1003

Web site: *http://www.ustoo.com*

This organization is an independent network of support group chapters for men with prostate cancer and their families. The organization offers a hotline that answers caller inquiries, provides literature, and makes referrals to its network of support groups. The web site provides information about prostate cancer, a listing of local support groups, clinical trials listing, online literature order form, newsletter articles, and many links to related sites. *Spanish materials are available.*

Y-ME National Breast Cancer Organization

212 W. Van Buren Street

Chicago, IL 60607

Toll-Free: 800-221-2141

Toll-Free (Spanish): 800-986-9505

Phone: 312-986-8338

Fax: 312-294-8597

Web site: *http://www.y-me.org*

This organization is a nonprofit organization serving men and women with breast cancer, as well as their families and friends. Y-ME has local chapters throughout the country. This organization offers a national hotline staffed by trained peer counselors who are breast cancer survivors (male and female), materials about breast health (including fibrocystic breast changes) and breast cancer monthly educational and support meetings throughout the country, information on comprehensive breast centers and treatment and research hospitals, referral to support groups nationwide, and wig and prosthesis banks. The web site offers information on the above services, general information on breast cancer and breast health, an electronic form to send questions to Y-ME staff, a list of publications, an electronic order form, and a list of Y-ME chapters. *Spanish-speaking staff and Spanish materials are available.*

HOME & HOSPICE CARE INFORMATION

Hospice Association of America (HAA)

228 Seventh Street, SE

Washington, DC 20003

Phone: 202-546-4759

Fax: 202-547-9559

Web site: *http://www.hospice-america.org*

This is a national trade association representing more than 2,800 hospices and thousands of caregivers and volunteers who serve terminally ill patients and their families. It is the largest lobbying group for hospice care, advocating the industry's interest before Congress, regulatory agencies, other national organizations, courts, media, and the general public. The HAA web site provides general information about hospice care, including a consumer's guide and a Bill of Rights for hospice patients.

Hospice Education Institute/Hospice Link

190 Westbrook Road
Essex, CT 06426
Toll-Free: 800-331-1620
Phone: 860-767-1620
Fax: 860-767-2746
Web site: *http://www.hospiceworld.org*

Hospice Link provides general information and materials about hospice care and makes referrals to local programs. It does not offer medical advice or personal counseling.

Hospice Foundation of America (HFA)

2001 S. Street, NW, Suite 300
Washington, DC 20009
Toll-Free: 800-854-3402
Phone: 202-638-5419
Fax: 202-638-5312
Web site: *http://www.hospicefoundation.org*

This organization offers information and materials on hospice care and educational programs. The HFA also maintains a current computerized directory of hospices and palliative care programs in the United States. The web site contains this information along with links to related sites.

Hospice Net

Web site: *http://www.hospicenet.org*

A nonprofit organization that works exclusively through on-line, Hospice Net provides articles regarding end-of-life issues. Hospice nurses, social workers, bereavement counselors, and chaplains are available to answer questions via e-mail. The web site includes information for patients and caregivers, information about grief and loss, and a hospice locator service.

National Association for Home Care (NAHC)

228 Seventh Street, SE
Washington, DC 20003
Phone: 202-547-7424

Fax: 202-547-3540

Web site: *http://www.nahc.org*

The NAHC provides a state-by-state database of phone numbers for home care and hospice agencies.

National Hospice and Palliative Care Organization

1700 Diagonal Road, Suite 300

Alexandria, VA 22314

Toll-Free Helpline: 800-658-8898

Fax: 703-525-5762

Web site: *http://www.nhpco.org*

This organization is dedicated to providing information about hospice care. The web site contains related links, a hospice locator database by state, a newsletter, and other general information.

Visiting Nurse Associations of America

11 Beacon Street

Boston, MA 02108

Toll-Free: 888-866-8773

Phone: 617-523-4042

Fax: 617-227-4843

Web site: *http://www.vnaa.org*

This organization's web site contains a visiting nurse locator, caregiver information, and related links to other organizations.

ORGANIZATIONS DEALING WITH FINANCIAL AND LEGISLATIVE ISSUES

Equal Employment Opportunities Commission

1801 L Street, NW

Washington, DC 20507

Toll-Free: 800-669-4000

Phone: 202-663-4900; 202-663-4494 (TDD)

Fax: 202-663-4912

Web site: *http://www.eeoc.gov*

This organization enforces federal statutes prohibiting employment discrimination. They offer information about statutes, employment discrimination, and

EEOC operations. Charges may be filed in person, by mail, or by phone. *Spanish-speaking staff are available.*

Health Insurance Association of America

555 13th Street, NW, Suite 600E

Washington, DC 20004

Toll-Free: 800-879-4422

Phone: 202-824-1600

Fax: 202-824-1722

Web site: *http://www.hiaa.org*

This organization represents most U.S. health insurance companies. It publishes a number of reports, manuals, and monographs, including an annual directory and an annual survey of hospitals.

Hill-Burton Hospital Care Program

Parklawn Building

5600 Fishers Lane, Room 10C-16

Rockville, MD 20854

Toll-Free: 800-638-0742

Phone: 301-443-5656

Fax: 301-443-0619

Web site: *http://www.hrsa.gov/osp/dfcr*

Hill-Burton is a government program whereby hospitals, nursing homes, and other medical facilities receiving funds from the government (usually for construction costs) are required by law to provide a reasonable amount of services to persons unable to pay. The Hill-Burton program web site contains a listing of Hill-Burton obligated facilities, eligibility criteria, and frequently asked questions. *Spanish materials are available.*

Internal Revenue Service (IRS)

Toll-Free: 800-829-1040

Toll-Free (for ordering publications): 800-829-3676

Web site: *http://www.irs.gov*

The IRS provides answers to tax questions, information about how to obtain tax forms and other publications, the status of an account or refund, and recorded information about tax laws. The IRS web site offers on-line publications and tax information, and electronic tax filing answers to frequently asked questions. *Spanish-speaking staff and Spanish materials are available.*

Office on the Americans with Disabilities Act

U.S. Department of Justice
Civil Rights Division
P.O. Box 66738
Washington, DC 20035-6738
Toll-Free: 800-514-0301; 800-514-0383 (TDD)
Phone: 202-301-0663
Fax: 202-307-1198

This office provides specific information about ADA requirements affecting public services and public accommodations. *Spanish-speaking staff and Spanish materials are available.*

National Association of Personal Financial Advisors

355 West Dundee Road, Suite 200
Buffalo Grove, IL 60089
Toll-Free: 888-333-6659
Phone: 847-537-7722
Fax: 847-537-7740
Web site: *http://www.napfa.org*

This organization serves as a network of full time, fee-only financial planners to discuss issues relating to practice management, client services, and investment selection. The organization provides referrals to certified financial planners by geographical area.

National Foundation for Consumer Credit (NFCC)

8611 Second Avenue, Suite 100
Silver Spring, MD 20910
Toll-Free: 800-388-2227
Toll-Free (Spanish): 800-682-9832
Phone: 301-589-5600
Fax: 301-495-5623

Web site: *http://www.nfcc.org*

The NFCC is a network of 1,450 nonprofit agencies that provide money management education, confidential budget, credit, and debt counseling, and debt repayment plans for both individuals and families. NFCC provides referrals to local consumer credit counseling services. The NFCC web site provides answers to frequently asked questions about bankruptcy, credit, and debt collection practices, information about how to obtain a credit report, and a directory of local NFCC member consumer credit counseling services.

American Alliance of Cancer Pain Initiatives (AACPI)
Resource Center

1300 University Avenue, Room 4720

Madison, WI 53706

Phone: 608-262-0978

Fax: 608-265-4014

Web site: *http://www.wisc.edu/trc; http://www.aacpi.org*

This organization promotes cancer pain relief by supporting the growth, development, and advocacy of State Cancer Pain Initiatives. The resource center offers a variety of education resources about pain management, such as patient education booklets and videos.

U.S. Department of Labor, Pension and Welfare Benefits Administration

200 Constitution Avenue, NW

Washington, DC 20210

Toll-Free: 800-998-7542

Phone: 202-219-8776

Fax: 202-219-8141

Web site: *http://www.dol.gov/dol/pwba*

This agency protects the integrity of pensions, health plans, and other employee benefits for more than 150 million people. This organization assists workers in protecting their benefit rights, assists benefit plan officials to understand the requirements of the benefit statutes, develops policies and laws that foster employment-based benefits, and deters and corrects violations of the relevant statutes. The Pension and Welfare Benefits Administration (PWBA) web site includes fact sheets on COBRA, ERISA, and HIPAA, questions and answers about recent changes in health care law, and information about employee benefit laws and regulations information on other PWBA programs. The Division of Technical Assistance and Inquiries assists the public with technical questions relating to pension, health, or other benefits offered by employers and protected by ERISA (Employment Retirement Income and Security Act of 1974), COBRA (the Consolidated Omnibus Budget Reconciliation Act of 1986), and HIPAA, (the Health Insurance Portability and Accountability Act of 1996).

Agency for Healthcare Research and Quality (AHRQ)

Publications Clearinghouse
P.O. Box 8547
Silver Springs, MD 20907-8547
Toll-Free: 800-358-9295
Fax: 301-594-2800
Web site: *http://www.ahrq.gov*

The AHRQ, an office within the U.S. Department of Health and Human Services, is responsible for supporting research designed to improve the quality of health care, reduce its cost, and broaden access to essential services. One of AHRQ's highest priorities is providing consumers with science-based, easily understandable information that will help them make informed decisions about their own personal health care. They offer a number of clinical practice guidelines on common health problems in consumer versions for the public. These guidelines are written by a panel of private-sector experts sponsored by AHRQ.

American Academy of Medical Acupuncture

58200 Wilshire Boulevard, Suite 500
Los Angeles, CA 90036
Toll-Free: 800-521-2262
Phone: 213-937-5514
Web site: *http://www.medicalacupuncture.org*

This organization is a professional organization that promotes the use of acupuncture by medical professionals. The organization provides a listing of medical health care providers who provide acupuncture treatment. All doctors are MDs or Doctors of Osteopathy. Callers can leave their name and address and a listing of professionals will be mailed to them. No other publications or services are available by phone. The web site includes information on acupuncture, acupuncturist locator that searches by specialty and area, contact information for schools of acupuncture worldwide, a listing of books and tapes that can be purchased.

American Brain Tumor Association

2720 River Road, Suite 146
Des Plaines, IL 60018
Toll-Free: 800-886-2282
Phone: 847-827-9910
Fax: 847-827-9918
Web site: *http://www.abta.org*

This is a nonprofit organization that supports research and promotes the understanding of brain tumors. They provide printed materials, an on-staff social worker, referrals to brain tumor support groups, a list of physicians participating in clinical trials, a pen-pal program, and a newsletter describing current research. The ABTA web site includes information about brain tumors and treatment, links to clinical trial databases, and text versions of the ABTA newsletter.

American Psychiatric Association

400 K Street, NW
Washington, DC 20005
Toll-Free: 888-357-7924
Fax: 202-682-6850
Web site: *http://www.psych.org*

This organization provides information on mental health and referrals.

American Psychological Association (APA)

750 First Street, NE
Washington, DC 20002-4242
Toll-Free: 800-374-2721
Phone: 202-336-5500
Web site: *http://www.apa.org*

This organization has a Division on Health Psychology that addresses a range of health issues including cancer. The APA provides a hotline to obtain literature and discuss psychological conditions, and referrals to state psychological associations to locate a psychologist in a specific area. The APA web site provides a help center with information about psychological issues. *Spanish-speaking staff are available.*

American Society for Clinical Hypnosis (ASCH)

33 West Grand Avenue, Suite 402
Chicago, IL 60610
Phone: 312-645-9810
Fax: 312-645-9818

This organization is a nonprofit society for health professionals interested in the clinical applications of hypnosis. Its purpose it to form and develop an organization of professional people in medicine, dentistry, nursing, psychology, social work, and mental health who share scientific and clinical interests in hypnosis. ASCH publishes pamphlets about hypnosis techniques and will provide a list of their members performing hypnosis in a specific geographical area if a self-addressed stamped envelope (business-size) is sent.

Joint Commission on Accreditation of Healthcare Organizations (JCAHO)

One Renaissance Boulevard
Oakbrook Terrace, IL 60181
Toll-Free (for filing complaints about a health care organization):
800-994-6610
Phone: 630-792-5000
Fax: 630-792-5005
Web site: *http://www.jcaho.org*

This is an independent nonprofit organization that evaluates and accredits more than 19,500 health care organizations in the United States, including hospitals, health care networks, and health care organizations that provide home care, long-term care, behavioral health care, laboratory, and ambulatory care services. JCAHO provides information to the public about accreditation status and selecting quality care. Performance reports of accredited organizations and guidelines for choosing a health care facility are available to the public and can be obtained by calling JCAHO or visiting their web site.

International Society of Psychiatric-Mental Health Nurses (ISPN)

1211 Locust Street
Philadelphia, PA 19107
Toll-Free: 800-826-2950
Fax: 215-545-8107
Web site: *http://www.ispn-psych.org*

The ISPN consists of specialty psychiatric-mental health nurses who treat patients with medical and mental health issues through counseling and education.

National Association of Social Workers

750 First Street NE, Suite 700
Washington, DC 20002-4241
Toll-Free: 800-638-8799
Phone: 202-408-8600
Fax: 202-336-8340
Web site: *http://www.naswdc.org*

This organization is concerned with advocacy, work practice standards and ethics, and professional standards for agencies employing social workers. The web site provides a national register of clinical social workers for local referrals. *Spanish-speaking staff are available.*

Oncology Nursing Society (ONS)

501 Holiday Drive
Pittsburgh, PA 15220-2749
Phone: 412-921-7373
Fax: 412-921-6565
Web site: *http://www.ons.org*

This organization is a national membership organization of registered nurses involved in oncology care whose mission is to promote professional standards for oncology nursing, research, and education. Nonmembers can access the ONS web site to find information about: cancer prevention, detection and screening, diagnosis, cancer treatment, survivorship, and-end-of life issues.

World Health Organization (WHO)

WHO Publications Center USA
49 Sheridan Avenue
Albany, NY 12210
Phone: 202-974-3000
Fax: 202-974-3663
Web site: *http://www.who.org*

The WHO is an agency of the United Nations which promotes technical cooperation for health among nations, carries out programs to control and eradicate disease, to control cancer pain, and strives to improve the quality of human life. The WHO web site includes data on numerous diseases and conditions, 2000 World Health Report, a list of publications, and links to related web sites. *Spanish materials are available.*

ADDITIONAL INTERNET

There is a vast amount of information about cancer on the Internet. This information can be very valuable to those facing cancer in making decisions about their illness and treatment. However, cancer information on the Internet can come from a variety of sources. Almost anyone can post information on the World Wide Web. While some may sound authoritative, the information may be inaccurate. Please consider the credentials and reputation of the organization providing the information. Always, discuss information you find on the Internet with your health care team. Internet information should not be a substitute for medical advice.

Association of Cancer Online Resources, Inc. (ACOR)

http://www.acor.org

This site contains an electronic mailing list that offers on-line support groups and cancer-related resources.

Center for Drug Evaluation and Research

U.S. Food and Drug Administration
http://www.fda.gov/cder

This government web site provides information about new drug development, over-the-counter drugs, and new drug approvals.

Centerwatch Clinical Trials Listing Service

http://www.centerwatch.com

This site offers a listing of industry and government sponsored clinical trials that are searchable by disease category. It also offers information on new drug therapies that have been approved by the FDA. Some helpful publications are also available.

HealthSCOUT

http://www.healthscout.com

This searchable site offers daily news and information on health topics.

OncoChat

http://www.oncochat.org

This site offers an on-line peer support group. It also has links to other on-line cancer resources Internet.

Quackwatch

http://www.quackwatch.com

This web site provides a guide to fraudulent claims about alternative medicines and questionable health products. The site is searchable by key word.

WebMD

http://my.webmd.com

This web site provides articles gathered from various sources (e.g., the ACS and the NCI) on a variety of health topics. The site is searchable by key word.

Additional Reading

While many of the agencies and organizations listed in this guide offer free pamphlets and booklets on cancer and related issues, there are several consumer books available that may also be of help.

AMERICAN CANCER SOCIETY PUBLICATIONS

Consumer Books

American Cancer Society. 2001. *A Breast Cancer Journey*. Atlanta, Ga.: American Cancer Society.

American Cancer Society. 2000. *American Cancer Society's Guide to Complementary and Alternative Cancer Methods*. Atlanta, Ga.: American Cancer Society.

Bostwick, D. G., G. T. MacLennan, and T. R. Larson. 1999. *Prostate Cancer: What Every Man—and His Family—Needs to Know*. Rev. ed. New York: Villard.

Eyre, H., D. Lange, and L. B. Morris. 2001. *Informed Decisions: The Complete Book of Cancer Diagnosis, Treatment, and Recovery, 2nd Edition*. Atlanta, Ga.: American Cancer Society.

Heiney, S., J. Hermann, K. Bruss, and J. Fincannon. 2001. *Cancer in the Family: Helping Children Cope with a Parent's Illness*. Atlanta, Ga.: American Cancer Society.

Houts, P., and J. Bucher. 2000. *Caregiving: A Step-By-Step Resource for Caring for the Person with Cancer at Home*. Atlanta, Ga.: American Cancer Society.

Levin, B. 1999. *Colorectal Cancer:* A Thorough and Compassionate Resource for Patients and Their Families. New York: Villard.

Runowicz, C. D., J. A. Petrek, and T. S. Gansler. 1999. *Women and Cancer: A Thorough and Compassionate Resource for Patients and Their Families*. New York: Villard.

Wilkes, G. M., T. B. Ades, and I. Krakoff. 2000. *Consumers Guide to Cancer Drugs*. Toronto: Jones & Bartlett.

Professional Books

Bast, R., D. Kufe, R. Pollock, R. Weichselbaum, J. F. Holland, and E. Frei, eds. 2000. *Cancer Medicine*. 5th Ed. Hamilton, Ontario: B.C. Decker, Inc. and the American Cancer Society.

Lauria, M., B. Clark, J. Hermann, and N. Stearns, eds. 2001. *Social Work in Oncology: Supporting Survivors, Families, and Caregivers.* Atlanta, Ga.: American Cancer Society.

Lenhard, Jr., R. E., R. T. Osteen, and T. Gansler, eds. 2001. *Clinical Oncology.* Atlanta, Ga.: American Cancer Society, 2001.

Petrek, J. A., P. I. Pressman, R. A. Smith, eds. 1998. *Lymphedema: Results From a Workshop on Breast Cancer Treatment-Related Lymphedema and Lymphedema Resource Guide.* Atlanta, Ga.: American Cancer Society.

Wilkes, G. M., T. B. Ades, and I. Krakoff. 1999. *Patient Education Guide to Oncology Drugs.* Boston: Jones & Bartlett.

Other Publications

Blum, L. 1992. *Free Money for Heart Disease and Cancer Care.* New York: Simon & Schuster.

Cancer Care. *A Helping Hand: The Resource Guide for People with Cancer.* 1998. Available from Cancer Care, Inc. at 800-813-4673 (*http://www.cancercare.org*).

Capossela, C., and S. Warnock. 1995. *Share the Care: How to Organize a Group for Someone Who is Seriously Ill.* New York: Fireside.

Cowles, J. 1993. *Pain Relief: How to Say No to Acute, Chronic & Cancer Pain!* New York: Mastermedia Limited.

Fromer, M. J. 1995. *Surviving Childhood Cancer: A Guide for Families.* Washington, D.C.: American Psychiatric Press.

Harpham, W. S. 1998. *After Cancer: A Guide to Your New Life.* Collingdale, Pa.: Diane Publishing.

Haylock, P. J., and C. P. Curtiss. 1997. *Cancer Doesn't Have to Hurt: How to Conquer the Pain Caused by Cancer and Cancer Treatment.* Salt Lake City, Utah: Hunter House.

Holland, J. C., and S. Lewis. 2000. *The Human Side of Cancer: Living with Hope, Coping with Uncertainty.* New York: HarperCollins.

Landay, D. 1998. *Be Prepared: The Complete Financial, Legal, and Practical Guide for Living with a Life-Challenging Condition.* New York: St. Martin's Press.

Lang S. S. and R. Patt. 1995. *You Don't Have to Suffer: A Complete Guide to Relieving Cancer Pain for Patients and Their Families.* New York: Oxford University Press.

Michigan State University. *Easing Cancer Pain* (CD-ROM). 1998. For details on obtaining single copies of the CD-ROM, contact the American Cancer Society, Michigan Division at 800-723-0360. A sample can be viewed at http://commtechlab.msu.edu/sites/cancerpain.

Morra, M., and E. Potts. 1994. *Choices: Required Reading for Anyone Facing Cancer.* Rev. ed. New York: Avon Books.

National Viator Representatives, Inc. *Every Question You Need to Ask Before Selling Your Life Insurance Policy.* Call 800-932-0050 for a free copy of the guide. Also available on-line at *http://www.nvrnvr.com.*

acupuncture. A technique in which very thin needles of varying lengths are inserted into the skin at specific points of the body to treat a variety of conditions, including pain.

acute pain. Pain that is severe, but lasts a relatively short time.

addiction. A psychological dependence on a medicine; uncontrollable drug craving, seeking, and use. Substance abusers, or addicts, take drugs to satisfy physical, emotional, and psychological needs—not to solve medical problems.

adjuvant analgesic. Medicine used in addition to primary cancer pain medicine.

adjuvant therapy. Treatment used in addition to the main treatment. It usually refers to hormonal therapy, chemotherapy, radiation therapy, or immunotherapy added after surgery to increase the chances of curing the disease or keeping it in check.

advance directives. Legal documents that tell the doctor and family what a person wants for future medical care, including whether to start or when to stop life-sustaining treatment.

alternative therapy. Use of an unproven therapy *instead of* standard (proven) therapy. Some alternative therapies have dangerous or even life-threatening side effects. With others, the main danger is that the patient may lose the opportunity to benefit from standard therapy. (*See* complementary therapy.)

analgesic. Medicine used to relieve pain.

anesthesia. The loss of feeling or sensation as a result of drugs or gases. General anesthesia causes loss of consciousness ("puts you to sleep"). Local or regional anesthesia numbs only a certain area.

anesthesiologist. A doctor who specializes in giving medicines or other agents that prevent or relieve pain, especially during surgery.

anticonvulsant. Medicine used to control seizures. Also used to control burning and tingling pain.

antidepressant. Medicine used to treat depression. Also used to treat tingling or burning pain from damaged nerves.

antiemetic. Medicine used to prevent or relieve nausea and vomiting.

antihistamine. Medicine used to control nausea and itching. Also used to help people sleep.

biofeedback. Treatment method that uses monitoring devices to help people consciously control certain body functions such as heartbeat, blood pressure, and muscle tension. This complementary nondrug method can help control pain.

biopsy. The removal of a sample of tissue to see whether cancer cells are present. In some, a very thin needle is used to draw fluid and cells from a lump.

brachytherapy. Internal radiation treatment given by placing radioactive material directly into the tumor or close to it. Also called *interstitial radiation therapy* or *seed implantation.*

breakthrough pain. A flare of pain that occurs when moderate to severe pain "breaks through" a regular pain medicine schedule used to control persistent pain or is felt for a short time.

catheter. A thin, flexible tube through which fluids enter or leave the body (e.g., a tube to drain urine).

central nervous system. Part of the body that includes the brain and spinal cord.

central venous catheter. A special thin, flexible tube placed in a large vein, usually in the chest or neck. It can remain there for as long as it is needed to deliver and withdraw fluids.

chemotherapy. Treatment with drugs to destroy cancer cells.

chronic pain. Pain that can range from mild to severe, and is present for a long time.

clinical trials. Studies of new treatments in patients. A clinical trial is only done when there is some reason to believe that the treatment being studied may be of value to the patient.

complementary therapy. Therapy used *in addition to* standard therapy. Some complementary therapies may help relieve certain symptoms of cancer, relieve side effects of standard cancer therapy, or improve a patient's sense of well being. (*See* alternative therapy.)

corticosteroid. Any of a number of naturally occurring or synthetically made substances used to reduce swelling and inflammation. Sometimes used as an anticancer treatment. (*See* steroid.)

distraction. A pain relief method, such as listening to music or using relaxation techniques, when you turn your attention to something other than the pain.

dose. The amount of medicine taken.

edema. Build-up of fluid in the tissues, causing swelling. Edema of the arm can occur after radical mastectomy, axillary dissection of lymph nodes, or radiation therapy. (*See* lymphedema.)

epidural. Injection of anesthetic drugs into the space around the sac that encloses the spinal cord.

fine needle aspiration. In this procedure, a thin needle is used to draw up (aspirate) samples for examination under a microscope. Also called FNA. (*See* biopsy.)

frequency. How often medicine is taken.

generic. Official name for a medicine, which describes the chemical content of the drug.

home health nurse. A nurse who visits a patient at home to assist with treatments or medications, teaches patients how to care for themselves, and assesses their condition to see if further medical attention is needed.

hospice. A special kind of care for people in the final phase of illness, their families, and caregivers. The care may take place in the patient's home, in a home-like facility, or within hospitals.

hypnosis. A state of restful alertness during which a person enters into a trance-like state, becomes more aware and focused, and is more open to suggestion.

imagery. Involves mental exercises that people use to think of pleasant images or scenes, such as waves hitting the beach, to help them relax.

immune system. The complex system by which the body resists infection by microbes such as bacteria or viruses and rejects transplanted tissues or organs. The immune system may also help the body fight some cancers.

incision. A cut made in the skin with a knife.

infusion. A method of giving pain medication into a vein through slow and/or prolonged delivery of a drug or fluid. Unlike an injection, which is given by a syringe, an infusion flows in by gravity or a mechanical pump.

injection. Using a syringe and needle to push fluids or drugs into the body; often called a "shot."

intra-arterial. Into an artery.

intramuscular (IM). Injection into a muscle.

intrathecal (IT). Injection into the spinal fluid.

intravenous (IV). A method of supplying fluids and medications using a needle inserted in a vein.

local anesthetic. A medicine that blocks the feeling of pain in a specific location in the body.

long-acting or sustained-release medicines. Medicines that work for long periods of time and that are taken at regular intervals during the day and night, such as oral analgesics that last twelve hours. (*See also* skin patch and transdermal.)

lymphedema. A complication that sometimes happens after breast cancer treatments. Swelling in the arm is caused by excess lymph fluid that collects after lymph nodes and vessels are removed by surgery or treated by radiation. This condition can be persistent but not painful.

medical oncologist. A doctor who is specially trained to diagnose and treat cancer with chemotherapy and other drugs.

metastasis. The spread of cancer from one part of the body to another.

narcotic. *See* opioid.

nerve block. A process to block pain by injecting pain medicine directly into or around a nerve or into the spine.

neurologist. A doctor specializing in the diagnosis and medical (non-surgical) treatment of nervous system diseases (i.e., diseases of the brain, nerves, and spinal cord).

neuropathic pain. A dull, burning sensation that can be caused by surgery.

neurosurgeon. A surgeon specializing in operations to treat nervous system disorders.

nonopioid. Medicine used for mild to moderate pain.

nonprescription pain medicine. Pain relief medicine (analgesics) that can be bought over-the-counter, without a doctor's order.

nonsteroidal anti-inflammatory drugs (NSAIDs). Medicines used to control mild to moderate pain and inflammation. They can be used alone or along with other medicines.

nurse practitioner. A registered nurse with an advanced degree. Licensed nurse practitioners diagnose and manage illness and disease, usually working closely with a doctor. In many states, they may prescribe medications.

oncologist. A doctor with special training in the diagnosis and treatment of cancer and symptoms of cancer.

oncology clinical nurse specialist. A registered nurse with a master's degree in oncology nursing who specializes in the care of cancer patients. Oncology clinical nurse specialists may prepare and administer treatments, monitor patients, prescribe and provide supportive care, and teach and counsel patients and their families.

oncology social worker. A person with a master's degree in social work who is an expert in coordinating and providing non-medical care to patients. The oncology social worker provides counseling and assistance to people with cancer and their families, especially in dealing with the non-medical issues that can result from cancer, such as financial problems, housing (when treatments must be taken at a facility away from home), and child care.

opioid. Medicine used for moderate to severe pain. Also known as a narcotic.

pain specialist. Oncologists, neurologists, anesthesiologists, neurosurgeons, and other doctors, nurses, or pharmacists who are experts in pain. A team of health professionals may also be available to address issues of pain control.

pain threshold. The point at which a person becomes aware of pain.

palliative care. Treatment to relieve, rather than cure, symptoms caused by cancer. Palliative care can help people live more comfortably.

palliative treatment. Treatment that relieves symptoms, such as pain, but is not expected to cure the disease. The main purpose is to improve the patient's quality of life.

pathologist. A doctor who specializes in diagnosis and classification of diseases by laboratory tests such as examination of tissue and cells under a microscope. The pathologist determines whether a tumor is benign or cancerous, and, if cancerous, the exact cell type and grade.

patient-controlled analgesia (PCA). A method that allows patients to control the administration of medicines at a rate and dosage that they choose.

persistent pain. Pain that is present for long periods of time, in most cases, all day long.

phantom limb pain. When a body part is removed during surgery, such as in a mastectomy or amputation, the person may still feel pain or other unpleasant sensations as if they were coming from the missing (phantom) part.

physical therapist. A health professional who uses exercises and other methods to restore or maintain the body's strength, mobility, and function.

physical therapy. A treatment used to regain the use of impaired muscles, increase range-of-motion in joints, relieve pain, and help perform activities of daily living. It involves exercise, electrical stimulation, hydrotherapy, and/or the use of massage, heat, cold, and electrical devices.

port. A small plastic or metal container surgically placed under the skin and attached to a central venous catheter inside the body. Blood and fluids can enter or leave the body through the port using a special needle.

primary care physician. The doctor a person would normally see first when a problem arises. A primary care doctor could be a general practitioner, a family practice doctor, a gynecologist, a pediatrician, or an internal medicine doctor (an internist).

prostaglandins. Substances naturally produced in the body and are present in many tissues.

psychiatrist. A medical doctor specializing in mental health and behavioral disorders. Psychiatrists prescribe medications and can also provide counseling.

psychologist. A licensed health professional (Ph.D., Psy.D., Ed.D.) who assesses a person's mental and emotional status and provides counseling.

radiation therapy. Treatment with high-energy rays (such as x-rays) to kill or shrink cancer cells. The radiation may come from outside of the body (external radiation) or from radioactive materials placed directly in the tumor (internal or implant radiation). Radiation therapy may be used to reduce the size of a cancer before surgery, to destroy any remaining cancer cells after surgery, or, in some cases, as the main treatment.

rapid-onset opioid. A medicine (opioid) used to relieve pain quickly.

rehabilitation. Activities used to help a person adjust, heal, and return to a full, productive life after injury or illness. This may involve physical restoration (such as the use of prostheses, exercises, and physical therapy), counseling, and emotional support.

relaxation techniques. Methods used to relieve pain or keep it from getting worse by reducing tension in the muscles.

short-acting medicines. Medicines that work quickly and stay in the body for short periods of time (also called "rescue" medicines).

side effect. An unintended symptom that results from using a drug or is an unwanted effect of treatment such as hair loss caused by chemotherapy, and fatigue caused by radiation therapy.

skin patch. A bandage-like patch that slowly releases medicine through the skin and then into the bloodstream. (*See* long-acting medicines and transdermal.)

skin stimulation. The use of pressure, friction, temperature change, or chemical substances to stimulate nerve endings in the skin. The feeling of pain can be lessened or blocked through skin stimulation.

steroid. Naturally occurring or synthetically made substance used to decrease swelling and inflammation.

subcutaneous infusion. Continuous delivery of medicines through a small needle implanted under the skin.

subcutaneous injection (SQ). Delivery of medicines by inserting a small needle beneath the skin.

suppository. A small solid substance, which is usually medicated, and inserted into various openings of the body, such as the rectum, vagina, or urethra, but not in the mouth. Once the suppository is inserted in the body it melts.

tolerance. When the body adjusts to a medicine so that either more medicine is needed to relieve pain or different medicine is needed.

Transcutaneous Electric Nerve Stimulation (TENS). A method of pain relief in which a special device transmits electrical impulses through electrodes to an area of the body that is in pain.

transdermal. A method using a bandage-like skin patch that releases medicine through the skin and into the blood stream. The medicine enters the body slowly and steadily. (*See* skin patch.)

viatical. The sale of a life insurance policy for cash.

Index

in children, 217–219, 224
counseling for, 288–289
pain and, 173
pain treatment and, 27–28
around-the-clock (ATC) schedule, 293
aspirin, 227
assets, 208
Association of Cancer Online Resources, Inc. (ACOR), 334
Association of Community Cancer Centers (ACCC), 313
autonomy, 249–251

ball of energy exercise, 154
bankruptcy, 211
bedsores, 43
biofeedback, 148–149, 223, 340
biopsy
cancer pain and, 29–30
definition, 340
bone marrow
anemia and, 103
aspiration, 30
bone pain, 41–42
brachytherapy, 101, 340
brand name medications
definition, 66
names of, 77
breads, 117
breakthrough pain. *See also* acute pain; chronic pain
controlling, 88
definition, 25, 282, 340
Brief Pain Inventory, 59–60
bronchoscopy, 31–32

Campaign Against Cancer, 246
Cancer Care, Inc., 318
Cancer Information and Counseling Line (CICL), 311
Cancer Information Service (CIS), 80, 316
cancer pain, 168–169. *See also* communication; complementary
nondrug treatments; drug therapy; pain assessment; pain
control
anticipating, 218–219
causes
bone marrow aspiration, 30
common, 282–283
diagnostic procedures, 28–33
endoscopy, 30–33
pain treatment, 34–40

tumor-related, 40–42
in children, 218–225
controlling, 144
definition, 23–24, 282
describing, 45–48, 220
in elderly patients, 225–230
emotional and social impact, 167–173
guidelines for pain management, 273–276
impact, 1–2
impact on relationships, 173–177
information resources, 311–317
intensity, 27–28, 48, 220, 231
misconceptions, 8–12
obstacles to relief, 283
other illnesses and, 42–43
psychosocial support services, 290
publications, 336–340
subjective nature of, 19–20
symptoms, 37
treatment guidelines, 295–305
types of, 24–27
undertreated, 2–3, 225, 230
Cancer Pain Treatment Guidelines for Patients, 279–305
Cancer Research Institute (CRI), 313
Cancer Survivors Network, 309–310
Cancer Trials, 315
CancerFax, 315
CANCERLIT (Bibliographic Database), 315
CancerNet, 315–316
Candlelighters Childhood Cancer Foundation (CCCF), 318
Candlelighters Foundation ombudsman program, 199
caregivers
communicating with, 17–18, 20–21, 48–51
for the elderly, 226
emotional reactions, 173
recommendations, 173
supervising medications, 231
categorical pain scale, 284–285
catheter, 223, 340
Center for Drug Evaluation and Research, 334
Centers for Disease Control and Prevention (CDC), 313
Centerwatch Clinical Trials Listing Service, 335
central nerve blocks, 110
central nervous system
confusion and delirium, 127–128
definition, 340
respiratory depression, 124–125
sedation, 125–127
central venous catheter, 341
cereals, 117

quality, of pain, 47

radiation oncologist, 16
radiation therapy
    definition, 288, 346
        palliative radiation therapy, 100–103
        side effects, 39–41, 102–103, 217
radical neck dissection, 36
radical nephrectomy, 36
radiopharmaceuticals, 101–103
range of motion exercises, 150–151
rapid-onset opioid medications, 346
Reach to Recovery program, 310–311
"reasonable accommodations" for disabled employees, 212
reassurance, 223
rectal suppositories, 82–83, 229, 292, 347
regional anesthesia, 222–223
registered nurses (RNs), 14–15
rehabilitation, 346
relationships, impact of cancer pain on, 173–177
relaxation, 157–159, 223, 288, 346
religious organizations, 206
"rescue" doses of opioids, 228
respiratory depression, 124–125
retirement plans, 207
Reverse Mortgage, 205
Reyes Syndrome, 222
rhythmic massage, 158
risk pools, 204–206

salivary glands, 102
scheduling medications, 293
sedation, 125–127
Selective Serotonin Reuptake Inhibitor (SSRI), side effects, 270
self-help groups, 179–180
severity, of pain, 27–28, 48
sexuality issues, 134–138
short-acting medications, 347
side effects
    adjuvant pain medicines, 267–272
    affecting the central nervous system, 124–128
    affecting the digestive tract, 114–119
    affecting the skin, 129–130
    anesthetic treatments, 79
    antianxiety drugs, 77
    anticonvulsants, 77, 268
    antidepressants, 77, 269–271
    antipyretic medications, 257

    antivomiting medications, 268
    chemotherapy, 37–39, 104, 217
    corticosteroids, 77, 79, 271–272
    definition, 347
    external beam radiation, 102
    managing, 75, 289–291
    nerve blocks, 109
    non-narcotics, 257
    NSAIDs, 72, 74, 120–124, 257–263
    opioid drugs, 113–128, 227–229, 263–266
    radiation therapy, 39–41, 102–103, 217
    radiopharmaceuticals, 102–103
    Selective Serotonin Reuptake Inhibitor (SSRI), 270
    tranquilizers, 78
    tricyclic antidepressants, 270–271
sigmoidoscopy, 31–33
silence, 221
simplified issue life insurance, 208
skin
    opioid drugs and, 129–130
    pressure sores, 43
skin patch, 82, 347–348. *See* transdermal medications
skin stimulation, 159–162, 348
skull, tumor-related pain, 41
slow rhythmic breathing exercises, 158
Social Security, 205
Social Security Administration, 323
Social Security Disability Income (SSDI), 201–202
social service organizations, 206
social worker, 16–17, 184
somatic pain, 283
spinal cord compression, 41
spinal opioid infusion, 111
spinal tap. *See* lumbar puncture
spirituality, 162–163
state laws. *See* legislative issues
state-sponsored plans, for uninsured patients, 204–206
steroids, 287, 348. *See also* corticosteroids
stiffness, 42–43
stimulants, for children, 222
stretching exercises, 150–151
subcutaneous (SQ or SC) injections, 84, 292, 347
sublingual medications, 82
substance abuse, 230–231
Supplemental Security Insurance (SSI), 191, 202, 205
support groups, 178–180
suppository, 82–83, 229, 292, 347
surgeon, 17
surgery
    cancer pain from, 34–37

cancer treatment, 288
  for children, 222
surrogate decision-maker, 251–253, 255
"sustained release" drugs, 69
sustained-release medications, 343
sympathetic nerve blocks, 110
synagogues, 206

T

Taking Charge of Money Matters, 193
Temporary Aid to Needy Families, 205
temporary nerve blocks, 107–108
TENS (transcutaneous electrical nerve stimulation), 163, 288, 347
terminal condition, definition, 242
terminal sedation, 238–239
thoracotomy, 36
Three-Step Analgesic Ladder for Cancer Pain Management, 67–68, 227, 275
thyroid gland, 102
tiredness, 139–141
titrated medications, 289
tolerance, 347
trade names. *See* brand name medications
tranquilizers, side effects, 78
transcutaneous electrical nerve stimulation (TENS), 163
transdermal medications, 82, 292, 347–348
transmucosal medications, 81–82
TRICARE, 201, 323
tricyclic antidepressants, side effects, 270–271
tumors
  cancer pain and, 40–42, 218
  treatment guidelines, 298–299

U

undertreated cancer pain, 2–3, 225, 230
uninsured patients, 204–206
urinary tract infections, 136
U.S. Department of Health and Human Services, 274, 330
U.S. Department of Labor
  Hotline on Women's Health and Cancer Rights Act, 213
  Wage and Hour Division, 213
U.S. Department of Labor, Pension, and Welfare Benefits Administration, 199, 329–330
U.S. Department of Veterans Affairs, 199, 201
U.S. Food and Drug Administration. *See* FDA
U.S. Social Security Administration, 199
US TOO International, 323

V

vaginismus, 136–137
vegetables, 117
Veterans Benefits, 203
veterans, insurance benefits for, 201
viatical loan, 209
viatical settlement, 209–210, 348
vibration, 161–162
visceral pain, 282
Visiting Nurse Associations of America, 326
visual analog scale, 57, 284–285, 303
visual concentration, 158
visualization, 153–155. *See also* imagery
vocational counseling, 214
vomiting, 118–120

W

WebMD, 335
Women's Health and Cancer Rights Act, 213
word scales, 57
workplace, legal protection, 211–214
World Health Organization (WHO)
  focus on pain control, ix
  guidelines for pain management, 275
  information resources, 334
  on pain treatment, 233
  on palliative care, 235–236
  Three-Step Analgesic Ladder for Cancer Pain Management, 67–68, 227, 275

Y

Y-ME National Breast Cancer Organization, 324
yoga, 164–165